"Loved your little book. It is ve... real data pronto. Anyone wh... basis would do well to get a copy of your book and re... is also wonderful as a reference."

Dr. Bruce West
Health Alert

"For years, I avoided cosmetics because of the fragrances or smothering effects I experienced when using them. ... Everyone concerned with looking good and being healthy needs this book to learn how to shop for cosmetics and health care products."

Ann P. Tidwell, Ph.D.
1st EnvrioSafety

"This handy book slips into my purse so nicely, I will never again shop for cosmetics or toiletries without it. Once again I am reminded that personal responsibility is the key to personal well being. Your book makes this job easier."

Barbara Van Horne, DC

"We love your ☺☺☺ system. We've been looking for a "non-biased" book on personal care products that's easy to follow and would allow us to assess products on our own by their ingredients. Your book is exactly what we were hoping to find."

Lisa Giordano, CNHP & Gregory Giordano, RN, CMT

"Your book is a truly useful reference guide. I've been checking labels since reading it and referencing back to your book. I never thought commercial toothpaste was particularly healthy, I just never realized before that it was a potentially deadly poison. It's in the wastebasket as is the can of shaving cream. And more, I'm sure, is yet to follow."

Bryan Stern, L.Ac.

"Finally! A compact, incredibly useful book that demystifies the labels on cosmetics. I have always hated the idea of putting toxic substances on my face--especially on my mouth and eyes--but labels never really helped me be a cautious consumer because the ingredients read like a foreign language. This book is a very valuable tool that I carry with me whenever I go shopping. Knowledge is power when it comes to fighting the battle against toxins. I love it!"

Stephanie Davis

Dying To Look Good:

The Disturbing Truth About What's Really in Your Cosmetics, Toiletries and Personal Care Products

Christine Hoza Farlow, D.C.

KISS For Health Publishing
"Keep It Simple Secrets For Health"

Every effort has been made to insure the accuracy of the
information in this book. However, nothing in this book
should be construed as medical advice or used in place of
medical consultation.

ISBN 0-9635635-3-X

To my husband David

and

my daughter Melissa.

Contents

How to Use This Book   11

Why You Should Use This Book   12

Buyer Beware   14

Safety Tips   16

Cosmetic Complaints   17

How the Classifications Were Determined   18

Cosmetic Ingredients   20

Choosing Safe Products   86

Makeup   89
    Foundations   89
    Face Powders   90
    Blushes   90
    Concealers   91
    Lipsticks, Glosses and Lip Pencils   92
    Eye Shadows   93
    Mascaras   94

Hair Care   95
    Shampoos   95
    Dandruff Shampoos   97
    Conditioners   97
    Women's Hair Coloring Products 102
    Men's Hair Coloring Products   102
    Hairsprays & Styling Products   102
    Men's Hairsprays & Styling Products   105

Dental & Oral Hygiene 106
    Toothpastes & Powders 106
    Mouthwashes 107

Feminine Hygeine 108
    Feminine Deodorants, Douches & Hygiene
    Preparations 108
    Tampons & Miscellaneous Menstrual
    Products 109

Nail Products 110
    Nail Polishes Hardeners & Protectors 110

Skin Products 111
    Deodorants & Antiperspirants 111
    Bath Oils, Bubble Baths & Mineral Baths 114
    Powders for Body Care 116
    Shaving Creams 116
    Skin Lotions 117
    Soaps 121

Outdoor Products 125
    Sunscreens 125
    Insect Repellants 125

Babies & Children 126
    Shampoos 126
    Conditioners 126
    Baby Powders 127
    Lotions and Creams 127
    Soaps 128
    Bubble Baths 128
    Toothpastes 128
    Sunscreen 128

Glossary 130

References 133

Dying To Look Good:

**The Disturbing Truth
About What's Really in
Your Cosmetics, Toiletries
and Personal Care Products**

HOW TO USE THIS BOOK

The codes below are to the left of each additive and indicate the safety of the additive when used for intended purposes in cosmetics and toiletries.

*   GRAS - <u>G</u>enerally <u>R</u>ecognized <u>A</u>s <u>S</u>afe by the FDA.

φ   FDA approved colorant

†   CIR (Cosmetic Ingredient Review) Expert Panel considers this ingredient safe

S   There is no known toxicity. The additive appears to be safe.

A   The additive may cause allergic reactions.

C   Caution is advised. The additive may be unsafe, poorly tested, or used in too many products we use on a regular basis.

C1   Caution is advised for certain groups in the population, such as pregnant women, infants, persons with high blood pressure, kidney problems, etc.

X   The additive is unsafe or very poorly tested.

Why You Should Use This Book

Your health is affected not only by what you put *into* your body in terms of food, drink, drugs and nutritional supplements, but also by what you put *on* your body. Your skin is not an impenetrable barrier as was thought years ago. We now know that all chemicals that come in contact with the skin can penetrate the skin in varying degrees. Many of the chemicals that can be absorbed through the skin have been detected in the blood stream.

Many of the ingredients used in cosmetics are toxic, even though they may not cause any reactions on the skin. Some even cause cancer. Some of the most commonly used ingredients combine with other ingredients to form cancer-causing substances. From 1978 to 1980, the FDA analyzed 300 cosmetic samples for carcinogenic contamination. Forty percent of the samples analyzed contained carcinogens. In 1991-92, they found that 65% of the cosmetic products sampled contained carcinogenic contaminants.

The cosmetics industry is very poorly regulated. The Federal Food, Drug, and Cosmetic (FD&C) Act does not require cosmetics or their ingredients to be approved before they are marketed and sold to consumers. FDA regulation starts *after* they are already in the marketplace. So, except for color additives and a few ingredients which are banned, manufacturers may use whatever ingredients they choose in the cosmetics they produce without approval from the FDA.

However, the Fair Packaging and Labeling Act requires cosmetic manufacturers to list the ingredients on the label of every cosmetic product sold directly to consumers in descending order of quantity. In other words, the ingredient present in the largest quantity appears first on the label and the ingredient present is the smallest quantity appears last.

Cosmetic manufacturers are not required to prove the claims

they make about their products or to test their products for safety. However, if the product's safety has not been established, the product requires the label to state: "WARNING: The safety of this product has not been determined."

This is not true, however, of hair coloring products, which are among the most poorly regulated consumer products. There is no requirement to place a warning on the label of hair coloring products to inform consumers that these products cause cancer. Using hair dye increases your risk for multiple myeloma, Hodgkin's disease, non-Hodgkins lymphoma and possibly breast cancer. There is strong evidence that as much as 20% of the cases of non-Hodgkins lymphoma in U.S. women may be a result of using hair dyes.

According to John Bailey, Ph.D., director of the FDA'S Office of Cosmetics and Colors, "Consumers believe that 'if it's on the market, it can't hurt me,' and this belief is sometimes wrong."

The FDA can make suggestions or recommendations to manufacturers about cosmetic products or their ingredients, but *the manufacturers do not have to comply*. The FDA must first prove in a court of law that a product is harmful, improperly labeled, or violates the law if it wants to remove a cosmetic product from the market.

The requirement to list cosmetic ingredients on the label applies to retail products sold for home use. Products produced for use in salons, labeled "For Professional Use Only" and cosmetic samples do not require the ingredients to be listed on the label. However, these products do require the name of the distributor, the quantity, and all necessary warning statements.

The Cosmetic, Toiletry and Fragrance Association (CTFA) International Buyers' Guide 1999 lists 25,854 cosmetic chemicals from which manufacturers can choose for the cosmetics they produce. Most of the chemicals have not been tested for short-term or long-term toxic effects or for systemic effects. Many are contaminated with toxic by-products from manufacturing. Many are toxic themselves.

The Cosmetic Ingredient Review (CIR), established in 1976 by CTFA, was an industry effort to provide an unbiased evaluation of the safety of cosmetic ingredients. Between 1976 and June 28, 2000, they completed safety assessments, on a priority basis, for 1018 ingredients. This represents only 3.9% of all the cosmetic ingredients in use.

In 1984, the National Research Council (NRC) identified 3,410 cosmetic ingredients as a potential public health hazard as part of the National Toxicology Program (NTP) to evaluate the need for chemical toxicity testing. As of mid 2000, almost 2400 of those chemicals still have not been tested, yet they continued to be used in cosmetic products.

Buyer Beware

The FDA's attempt at establishing official definitions for specific terms like "natural" and "hypoallergenic" were overturned in court. Consequently, companies can use these terms on cosmetic labels to mean anything they want. Mostly, the value of these terms lies in promoting cosmetic products to the consumer rather than any real medical meaning, according to dermatologists.

Beware of products claiming to be:

- Natural – this suggests that the ingredients are derived from natural sources rather than being produced synthetically. However, there are no standards for what natural means. The product may contain all natural ingredients, just a few natural ingredients added to a synthetic product, or even no natural ingredients at all.

- Hypoallergenic – this means that the manufacturer believes the product is *less likely* to cause allergic reactions. But there are no standards for classifying a product hypoallergenic. The manufacturer may actually test the product before classifying it hypoallergenic, or simply remove fragrances and call it hypoallergenic. The manufacturer is not required to prove this claim. Also, the terms "dermatologist-tested," "sensitivity tested," "allergy tested," or "nonirritating" do not guarantee they won't cause allergic reactions.

- Alcohol Free – this generally means the product does not contain ethyl alcohol (or grain alcohol). The product may contain fatty alcohols like cetyl, cetearyl, stearyl, or lanolin.

- Fragrance Free – this means that the product has no detectable odor. Fragrance ingredients may still be added to mask offensive odors from the materials used to make the product.

- Noncomodogenic – this implies that there are no pore-clogging ingredients that may cause acne in the product.

- Cruelty Free – this suggests that there has been no animal testing of the product. In reality, the majority of cosmetic ingredients have been tested on animals at some point. A more accurate statement would be "no new animal testing," if indeed this were the case.

- Shelf Life (Expiration Date) – this gives the length of time a cosmetic product is good if handled and stored properly. Expiration dates are approximate, and in reality,

15

a product may expire long before the expiration date.

Safety Tips

Here are a few tips to help you use your cosmetics safely and protect yourself from harm associated with the misuse of cosmetics.

- Never apply makeup while driving. An accidental scratch to your eyeball can cause bacterial infection and result in serious injury, including blindness.

- Never share makeup.

- Be wary of testers at cosmetics counters. They may be contaminated. If you must test before purchasing, insist on a new disposable applicator and that the salesperson clean the container opening with alcohol and before applying to your skin.

- Never add liquid to a cosmetic product to restore its original consistency. This may cause bacterial contamination.

- Stop using a product if you've had an allergic reaction to it.

- Throw away products in which there has been a change in color or odor.

- Do not use eye makeup if you have an eye infection. Discard all products you were using when you discovered the infection.

- Keep makeup out of sunlight.

- Close makeup containers tightly when not in use.

- Many aerosol products are flammable. Do not use near heat or while smoking. Do not inhale hairsprays and powders. They may cause lung damage.

Cosmetic complaints

The FDA maintains the Cosmetic Adverse Reaction Monitoring Database to keep track of adverse reactions to cosmetics. The FDA estimates, however, that it receives only a small percentage of complaints about cosmetics filed by consumers. Poison control centers, manufacturers and distributors, and state and local agencies are more likely to receive complaints of adverse reactions to cosmetics.

The most common complaints reported to the FDA in 1999 were related to dermatitis, fragrance sensitivity, nervous system reactions, pain, respiratory system reactions, and tissue damage.

If you experience adverse reactions to cosmetics, you can report it to:

> Food and Drug Administration
> Center for Food Safety and Applied Nutrition
> Office of Colors and Cosmetics
> 200 Street, SW
> Washington, DC 20204
> (202) 205-4494

How the Classifications Were Determined

Many references were used in determining how to classify
each ingredient in this book according to safety. In addition to
the references listed in the back of the book, available
information was reviewed from the

- Cosmetic Ingredient Review (CIR)
- National Fire Protection Association (NFPA) Chemical
  Hazard Ratings
- National Toxicology Program (NTP) Report on
  Carcinogens
- International Agency for Research on Cancer (IARC)
- Material Safety Data Sheets (MSDS) from chemical
  manufacturers and various government agencies.

In many cases, the various references were not in complete
agreement as to the safety of the ingredient. In those cases, I
have taken the conservative approach: if there is any
indication from any of the sources that the ingredient might
have any adverse effects, then they were noted and rated
according to the significance or severity of the adverse
reactions. In most cases, the references indicating the most
severe reactions were given the most weight.

All ingredients that are known carcinogens are rated X or
unsafe. Ingredients that are not carcinogenic, but are known to
be unsafe for various reasons, are also rated X. Ingredients
that are not themselves carcinogenic, but may potentially form
a carcinogen when they react with another ingredient in the
product are rated C or caution. Ingredients that are not
carcinogenic, but may be contaminated with a carcinogen in
the production of the ingredient are also rated C. In addition,
ingredients that may cause a variety of mild to moderate
adverse effects are rated C.

Ingredients that may have some harmful effects for certain
groups of the population are rated C1 and the affected groups

are noted. For example, an ingredient may have some adverse effects for children or pregnant women.

In some cases, the ingredients may be rated S or safe and have some adverse reactions listed. In these cases, based upon known information, the ingredient is considered basically safe, but under certain conditions, which may be avoidable, they may cause a reaction. For example, an ingredient may cause photosensitivity if you go out into the sun after using a product containing the ingredient, but if you wait a few hours before going out in the sun or if you avoid the sun, there is no reaction. Or the ingredient is considered basically safe for the general population, but a very few people may have a mild reaction to the ingredient.

The safest products are products with the fewest number of ingredients and with the ingredients rated S. However, even if all of the ingredients used in our cosmetics and personal care products are safe individually, rarely does any product have only one ingredient in it. Testing for ingredient safety has only been done for individual ingredients, not for combinations of ingredients. Ingredients that are safe individually may be harmful in certain combinations. Nobody knows the effects of the many different ingredients used in the thousands of different combinations.

Cosmetic Ingredients

S   <u>Abies alba</u> – see fir oil.

S   <u>Abies sibirica</u> – see fir oil.

C   <u>Acetic ether</u> - see ethyl acetate.

X   <u>Acetone</u> – eye, nose, throat and skin irritant; may cause light headedness, nausea, coma, nail splitting, peeling and brittleness; lung irritant if inhaled; narcotic in large amounts; neurotoxin; has caused liver, kidney, and nerve damage in lab animals; extremely toxic.

X   <u>Acetophenetidide</u> – see phenacetin.

X   <u>Acetophenetidin</u> – see phenacetin.

X   <u>Acetyl ethyl tetramethyl tetralin</u> - toxic to nervous system, may cause hyperirritability; has caused brain, spinal cord and nervous system damage and death in lab animals; absorbs through the skin.

†CA   <u>Acetylated lanolin</u> - skin irritant; may cause acne; see lanolin.

S   <u>Achillea millefolium</u> – see yarrow oil.

X   <u>Acid Blue 9</u> – coal tar dye; carcinogen.

S   <u>Aesculus hippocastanum</u> - herb, anti-inflammatory, for sensitive skin, capillary fragility.

X   <u>AETT</u> – see acetyl ethyl tetramethyl tetralin.

C   <u>Alcohol</u> - can cause contact dermatitis; see ethyl alcohol.

S   <u>Alcohol C12</u> - see lauryl alcohol.

C   <u>Alkaline persulphates</u> – has caused asthma in hairdressers; contains ammonium salts, see ammonia.

CA   <u>Alkanoamides</u> - may cause formation of carcinogenic nitrosamines in products containing nitrogen compounds; cause contact dermatitis.

C   <u>Alkoxylated alcohols</u> - may contain dangerous levels of toxins.

C   <u>Alkoxylated amides</u> - may cause formation of carcinogenic nitrosamines in products containing nitrogen compounds; cause contact dermatitis.

C   <u>Alkoxylated amines</u> - may contain dangerous levels of toxins; see amines.

C   <u>Alkoxylated carboxylic acids</u> - may contain dangerous levels of toxins.

C   <u>Alkyl ether sulfates</u> - may cause formation of carcinogenic nitrosamines in products containing nitrogen compounds; cause contact dermatitis; contains ammonium salts, see ammonia.

C   <u>Alkyl sulfates</u> - may cause dermatitis, irritate skin; contains ammonium salts, see ammonia.

S   <u>Allantoin</u> – herb; healing properties; may irritate skin.

S   <u>Allium sativum</u> - herb, see garlic.

SA   <u>Almond glycerides</u> – potential skin irritant.

SA   <u>Almond oil</u> – carrier oil; healing for irritated or dry skin; may irritate skin.

S   <u>Aloe</u> - herb, healing properties; antibacterial; anti-inflammatory; moisturizer.

S   <u>Aloe extract</u> – see aloe, extract.

S   <u>Aloe vera</u> – see aloe.

S   <u>Aloe vera gel</u> – see aloe.

S   <u>Aloe vera juice</u> – see aloe.

S   <u>Alpha-bisabolol</u> – herb; component of chamomile; non-allergenic; anti-inflammatory.

†C   <u>Alpha hydroxy acids</u> – causes photosensitivity which subsides within a week of discontinuing use; penetrates skin more deeply in cream base; safety of long-term use unknown; CIR panel says safe if concentration is 10% or less, pH is 3.5 or greater, and product is formulated so it protects the skin from increased sun sensitivity or tells consumer to use sun protection.

C   <u>Alpha-hydroxytoluene</u> - may cause contact dermatitis.

C   <u>Alpha-methylquinoline</u> - skin irritant; see quinaldine.

C   <u>Alpha-pinene</u> - irritates skin, may cause contact dermatitis.

S   <u>Althea extract</u> – see marshmallow, extract.

S   <u>Althea officinalis</u> – see marshmallow.

21

CA   <u>Aluminum chloride</u> – skin irritant; moderately toxic if swallowed.

CA   <u>Aluminum chlorohydrate</u> – skin irritant; may cause hair follicle infections.

CA   <u>Aluminum phenolsulfate</u> – skin irritant; contains ammonium salts, see ammonia, aluminum sulfate.

*CA   <u>Aluminum sulfate</u> – skin irritant; moderately toxic if swallowed; not shown to be safe; ammonium salt, see ammonia.

φC   <u>Aluminum powder</u> – may be causative factor in Alzheimer's; inhalation can cause lung disease; see external use only.

C   <u>Amines</u> - may cause formation of carcinogenic nitrosamines in products containing nitrogen compounds; cause contact dermatitis.

C   <u>Amino acids</u> – components of protein necessary for health; may contain hidden MSG; see MSG.

C   <u>2-aminoethanol</u> - see ethanolamine.

†CA   <u>Aminoform</u> - see methenamine.

†X   <u>2-amino-4-nitrophenol</u> – skin irritant; may cause convulsions with skin contact; may cause asthma if inhaled; sensitizer; mutagen, may cause genetic damage.

†X   <u>2-amino-5-nitrophenol</u> – see 2-amino-4-nitrophenol.

†X   <u>4-amino-2-nitrophenol</u> – see 2-amino-4-nitrophenol.

†C   <u>Aminomethyl propanol</u> – may irritate skin; used in concentrations up to 10%; not adequately tested for concentrations exceeding 1%; CIR panel says safe in concentrations up to 1%.

XA   <u>Ammonia</u> – corrosive; toxic if inhaled; eye and mucous membrane irritant; can burn eyes and skin; can cause permanent damage; classified as hazardous by OSHA; best to avoid all cosmetics containing ammonia or ammonium salts.

CA   <u>Ammonia water</u> – mucous membrane and eye irritant; may blister and burn skin; toxic when inhaled; see ammonia.

XA   <u>Ammoniated mercury</u> – skin irritant; can be absorbed through the skin and cause poisoning; may cause kidney damage; toxic; see ammonia.

XA   Ammonium chloride – severe eye and skin irritant; toxic if ingested in large amounts; may cause irreversible damage; see ammonia.

CA   Ammonium hydroxide – severe skin, eye and mucous membrane irritant; poison when swallowed in large amounts; can burn the skin and cause hair to break; see ammonia.

†CA   Ammonium laureth sulfate – mild irritant; may be contaminated with carcinogenic 1,4-dioxane; see ethoxylated alcohols, ammonia.

†CA   Ammonium lauroyl sarcosinate - CIR panel says safe in "rinse-off" products, safe at 5% concentrations in "leave-on" products, insufficient data to determine safety in products which might be inhaled, may cause formation of carcinogens in products containing nitrogen compounds; see ammonia.

†CA   Ammonium lauryl sulfate – mild irritant; for brief skin contact only, rinse thoroughly; CIR panel says safe in "rinse-off" products and up to 1% concentrations in "leave-on" products; see ammonia.

†CA   Ammonium thioglycolate – cumulative severe skin irritant; may cause burns and blisters; sensitizer; CIR panel says can be used infrequently at concentrations up to 14.4%, see ammonia.

XA   Ammonium xylenesulfonate – not adequately tested; see ammonia, xylene.

C   Amorphous hydrated silica – respiratory, eye and skin irritant; may be contaminated with crystalline quartz, a carcinogen; see external use only.

C   Amorphous fumed silica – respiratory, eye and skin irritant; may be contaminated with crystalline quartz, a carcinogen; see external use only.

C   Amphoteric-2 – gentle cleanser; petroleum based; composed of betaines and imidazoles; imidazole is a benzene derivative, but is an inhibitor rather than a toxin; see benzene.

C Amphoteric-6 – see amphoteric-2.

C Amphoteric-20 – see amphoteric-2.

S Aniba roseodora – see rosewood.

S Anise oil - essential oil; may cause dermatitis; see essential oils.

C Anionic surfactants – may be contaminated with carcinogenic nitrosamines; highly absorbable through skin, even in "rinse-off" products.

X o-anisidine – sensitizer; skin irrritant; absorbed through skin; possible carcinogen.

φS Annatto

X Anthanthrene – carcinogen; mineral oil contaminant.

S Anthemis nobilis - essential oil; antiallergenic; antibacterial; anti-inflammatory; astringent; healing for skin; potential sensitive skin irritant.

S Apricot oil – carrier oil; moisturizing.

C1 Arctium lappa – herb; antibacterial; antidandruff; astringent; avoid if pregnant.

C1 Artemesia dracunculus – see tarragon oil.

S Artemisia pallens – see davana.

C1 Asafetida – possible irritant if chemically sensitive; infants and young children should avoid.

*SA Ascorbic acid - synthetic vitamin C; one component of the vitamin C complex; see nutrient additives; can enhance mineral absorption, can inhibit nitrosamine formation; may be corn based.

†S Avocado oil – carrier oil.

C Azulene - see guaiazulene.

S Balm – see melissa oil.

CA Balsam of Peru – skin irritant; causes contact dermatitis; sensitizer.

C Barium –skin, eye and respiratory irritant; never use on broken skin; poisonous if ingested; see external use only.

*SA Bay oil – essential oil; skin irritant.

†S Beeswax – skin irritant.

XA Benzaldehyde – gastrointestinal, mucous membrane, eye and skin irritant; central nervous system depressant; large doses cause convulsions, poisoning; highly toxic.

†XA   Benzalkonium chloride – eye and skin irritant; extremely toxic; CIR says this is safe in concentrations up to .1%; some products contain up to 5%; see quaternary ammonium compounds.

C   Benzamidines - may cause contact dermatitis, skin irritation.

X   Benzene – petroleum based; skin and mucous membrane irritant; absorbed through skin; photosensitizer; poison if ingested; causes aplastic anemia, poisoning of bone marrow; may cause leukemia; banned in numerous household products; carcinogen.

CA   Benzenecarboxylic acid - skin irritant, harmful if ingested.

X   Benzo-a-pyrene – carcinogen; mineral oil contaminant.

X   Benzo-b-fluroanthene – carcinogen; mineral oil contaminant.

C   Benzoates - may cause contact dermatitis.

CA   Benzocaine - may cause contact dermatitis, has caused oxygen loss in the blood of babies, central nervous system irritability in adults.

†CA   Benzoic acid - skin irritant, harmful if ingested; CIR panel says safe in concentrations up to 5%, insufficient data to support safety in products where exposure involves inhalation.

C   Benzoic acid ethyl ester - see ethyl benzoate.

C   Benzoic ether - see ethyl benzoate.

SA   Benzoin - antiseptic, anti-inflammatory; may irritate sensitive skin, cause drowsiness; if diluted in solvent instead of alcohol, solvents may be absorbed into the bloodstream; solvents are toxic.

SA   Benzoin balm - essential oil; see benzoin.

SA   Benzoin oil - essential oil; see benzoin.

CA   Benzoin tincture – see benzoin, ethyl alcohol.

†C   Benzophenone-n (1-12) - may cause extreme contact

dermatitis, photosensitivity.

CA   <u>Benzopyrone</u> - see coumarin.

CA   <u>Benzoyl peroxide</u> – skin irritant and allergen; toxic if inhaled.

†C   <u>Benzyl alcohol</u> – severe eye, moderate skin and mucous membrane irritant; poison if ingested; CIR panel says safe in concentrations up to 5%, up to 10% in hair dyes, insufficient data to support safety in products where exposure involves inhalation.

C A   <u>Benzyl benzoate</u> - skin and eye irritant.

C   <u>Benzylparaben</u> - preservative, may cause mild irritation; insufficient data to support safety according to CIR panel.

*CA   <u>Bergamot oil</u> - essential oil; antibacterial, antiperspirant, astringent, healing properties for hair and skin; may cause contact dermatitis; photosensitizer; see essential oils.

φS   <u>Beta carotene</u> - vitamin A precursor; antioxidant.

C1A   <u>Betula alleghaniensis</u> – see birch oil.

CA   <u>Betula pendula</u> – herb; healing to skin; see birch oil.

X A   <u>BHA</u> - may cause contact dermatitis; harmful if ingested; can cause liver and kidney damage, behavioral problems, infertility, weakened immune system, birth defects; should be avoided by infants, young children, pregnant women, those sensitive to aspirin; possible carcinogen.

X A   <u>BHT</u> - similar to BHA, but more toxic; banned in England.

C   <u>Bilberry</u> – herb; anti-inflammatory; for sensitive skin, gingivitis; may interfere with iron absorption; avoid long-term use; use for 3 weeks periods then take a break.

S   <u>Biotin</u> - important for hair and skin; see nutrient additives.

CA   <u>Birch</u> – herb; see birch oil.

CA   <u>Birch oil</u> - essential oil; avoid if pregnant, epileptic or aspirin sensitive; see methyl salicylate.

S   <u>Bisabolol</u> - see alpha-bisabolol.

XA   Bismuth - may cause memory loss, intellectual impairment, nervous system disorders; poison.

φCA   Bismuth citrate – poison; absorbed through skin; approved for hair dyes only up to .5% concentration; see bismuth.

φCA   Bismuth oxychloride – skin irritant; low toxicity in cosmetics; see bismuth.

S   Blue mallow – herb; antiallergenic; anti-inflammatory; for sensitive skin.

φXA   Blue No. 1 – see FD&C Blue No. 1.

XA   Blue No. 1 Lake – see FD&C Blue No. 1 Lake.

XA   Blue No. 2 – see FD&C Blue No. 2.

XA   Blue No. 2 Lake – see FD&C Blue No. 2 Lake.

C   Blue No. 99 - may cause contact dermatitis.

X A   Boranes – extremely toxic, may cause contact allergies.

†C   Boric acids - suspected toxin; topical and internal use have caused poisonings; do not use on infants or damaged skin; CIR panel says safe up to 5% concentration.

CA   Bornelone - may cause contact dermatitis.

S   Boswellia carterii – see frankincence oil.

†C   2-bromo-2-nitropropane-1,3-diol - see bronopol.

†C   Bronopol – toxic; causes contact dermatitis, may cause the formation of carcinogenic nitrosamines; may break down into formaldehyde, a probable carcinogen; see formaldehyde.

φS   Bronze powder – flammable.

C1   Burdock – see arctium lappa.

†C   Butane – propellant in aerosol products; petroleum derivative; flammable; may cause drowsiness, asphyxiation; mildly toxic if inhaled; neurotoxic in high doses.

CA   Butanol - see butyl alcohol.

†CA   Butyl acetate – petroleum derivative; toxic; irritant to skin and respiratory tract; central nervous system depressant.

CA   Butyl alcohol - petroleum derivative; skin, eye and
        respiratory irritant; may cause liver damage.
X   Butyl Cellosolve – petroleum derivative; used in hair
        dyes; poison; eye and skin irritant; highly absorbable
        through skin; neurotoxin.
CA   Butyl octadecanoate - petroleum derivative; may
        cause acne.
SA   Butyl stearate - petroleum derivative; may cause
        acne.
X A   Butylated hydroxyanisole - petroleum derivative; see
        BHA.
X A   Butylated hydroxytoluene - petroleum derivative; see
        BHT.
XA   Butylene glycol – petroleum derivative; see ethylene
        glycol.
XA   Butylhydroxyanisol - petroleum derivative;
        carcinogen.
CA   Butylparaben - petroleum derivative; skin irritant.
SA   Cacao butter - see cocoa butter
X   Cadmium chloride – used in hair dyes; carcinogen;
        ingestion can be fatal.
C   Cajaput oil - essential oil; antibacterial, anti-
        inflammatory; skin irritant; may cause internal
        bleeding and vomiting if taken internally; use with
        caution; see essential oils.
C   Cajeput oil - see cajaput oil.
*C   Calcium carbonate – moderate to severe skin and eye
        irritant.
C   Calcium oxide – severe mucous membrane and skin
        irritant; may cause chemical burns.
S   Calendula – herb; soothes inflammation; may cause
        dermatitis.
S   Calendula extract - see calendula, extract.
S   Calendula officinalis – see calendula.
S   Canagium odoratum - see ylang ylang oil.
S   Cananga odorata – see ylang ylang oil.
S   Canarium luzonicum – see elemi oil.
X   Canthanaxin – effects on the human body are

unknown; not adequately tested.

X   <u>Canthaxanthin</u> - ingestion can cause night blindness, aplastic anemia; has caused death

C   <u>Canola oil</u> – may be genetically modified.

φS   <u>Caramel</u>

C1   <u>Caraway oil</u> - essential oil; promotes wound healing; external use only; caution if pregnant.

C   <u>Carba-mix</u> - may cause contact dermatitis.

*C   <u>Carbamide</u> – see urea.

X   <u>3-carbethoxypsoralen</u> - phototoxic chemical, may damage DNA and cause mutations, tumors or neoplasms.

X   <u>Carbitol</u> – toxic.

CA   <u>Carbomer</u> – eye, skin, respiratory and digestive tract irritant; not adequately tested.

CA   <u>Carbomer 934</u> – see carbomer.

CA   <u>Carbomer 940</u> – see carbomer.

CA   <u>Carbomer 941</u> – see carbomer.

CA   <u>Carboxobenzene</u> - skin irritant, harmful if ingested.

C   <u>Carboxymethyl cellulose</u> – has caused cancer, birth defects, sterility, infertility in animals when ingested; skin toxicity unknown.

φCA   <u>Carmine</u> – derived from dried insects; may irritate skin in sensitive individuals; may cause hives; when ingested has caused hives, asthma and anaphylactic shock.

S   <u>Carotene</u> - see beta carotene.

*C   <u>Carrageenan</u> – possible carcinogen.

S   <u>Carrot extract</u> - may cause photo sensitivity.

S   <u>Carrot oil</u> – essential oil; healing to the skin; see essential oils.

C1   <u>Carum carvi</u> – see caraway oil.

CA   <u>Caryophyllus oil</u> - see clove oil

S   <u>Castile soap</u>

CA   <u>Castor oil</u> - toxic if ingested; eye irritant; may cause allergic cheilitis.

C1   <u>Cedarwood oil</u> – essential oil; astringent, antifungal, antibacterial; use cautiously or avoid if pregnant; see essential oils.

C1   <u>Cedrus atlantica</u> – see cedarwood oil.

C   <u>Cedrus virginiana</u> – astringent; antifungal; antibacterial; avoid if pregnant; potentially toxic; use small amounts.

C1   <u>Centella asiatica</u> – see gotu kola.

SA   <u>Centrurea cyanus</u> – herb; causes photosensitivity.

SA   <u>Ceresin</u> – petroleum derivative.

SA   <u>Ceresine* Earth Wax</u> – petroleum derivative.

†S   <u>Cetearyl alcohol</u> - may cause contact dermatitis.

C   <u>Ceteth-n</u> - may contain dangerous toxic byproducts; see ethoxylated alcohols.

†C   <u>Cetrimonium bromide</u> – skin and eye irritant; sensitizer; fatal if swallowed; teratogen in mice; CIR panel says safe in "rinse-off" products and up to .25% concentrations in "leave-on" products.

SA   <u>Cetyl alcohol</u> - may cause skin irritation.

C   <u>Cetyl stearyl alcohol</u> - may cause contact dermatitis.

†SA   <u>Cetylic acid</u> - see palmitic acid.

SA   <u>Cetylic alcohol</u> - may cause skin irritation.

X   <u>Chinaldine</u> – skin irritant; see quinaldine.

SA   <u>Chamomile</u>- herb; anti-inflammatory; may cause allergic contact dermatitis.

SA   <u>Chamomile blossom extract</u> – soothing for bruises and inflammation; see chamomile.

SA   <u>Chamomile extract</u> – see chamomile, extract.

C1A   <u>Chamomile oil</u> - essential oil; antibacterial, anti-inflammatory, astringent, healing for skin; may irritate sensitive skin; use cautiously if pregnant; see essential oils.

C   <u>Chinese anise</u> - essential oil is toxic; herb should be used very sparingly.

CA   <u>Chinese cinnamon oil</u> - essential oil; avoid if pregnant or fever.

X   <u>Chloroacetamide</u> – CIR panel determined this ingredient to be unsafe.

CA   <u>Chloracetamide</u> - skin, eye and mucous membrane irritant; can be fatal if swallowed.

X	<u>Chloramphenicol</u> - antibiotic; may cause eczema; hazardous side effects; probable carcinogen.
X	<u>Chlorofluorocarbons</u> – carcinogen; banned in aerosol products in the US.
C	<u>Chloromethylisothiazolinone</u> - may cause contact dermatitis.
CA	<u>5-chloro-2-methyl-4-iso thiazolin-3-one</u> – see isothiazolinones.
CA	<u>5-chloro-3-methyl isothiazolone</u> - can cause contact allergies.
X	<u>4-chloro-1,2-phenylenediamine</u> – carcinogen.
X	<u>4-chloro-o-phenylenediamine</u> – carcinogen.
X	<u>2-chloro-p-phenylenediamine sulfate</u> – carciniogen; contains ammonium salts, see ammonia.
φS	<u>Chlorophyllin-copper complex</u> – see potassium sodium copper chlorophyllin.
C	<u>Chloropromazine group</u> - causes phototoxicity.
C	<u>Choleth-n</u> - may contain dangerous levels of toxic byproducts; see ethoxylated alcohols.
CA	<u>Chromates</u> - may cause contact dermatitis.
φCA	<u>Chromium hydroxide green</u> – irritant if inhaled; severe gastrointestinal irritant if ingested; long-term exposure may cause cancer; see external use only.
φCA	<u>Chromium oxide greens</u> – see chromium hydroxide green.
*CA	<u>Cinnamal</u> – see cinnamic aldehyde.
*CA	<u>Cinnamaldehyde</u> - see cinnamic aldehyde.
CA	<u>Cinnamate</u> - may cause skin rashes.
CA	<u>Cinnamic acid</u> - see cinoxate.
*CA	<u>Cinnamic aldehyde</u> – gastrointestinal, mucous membrane and skin irritant; may cause depigmentation; toxic if swallow large amounts.
CA	<u>Cinnamomum verum</u> – see cinnamon bark oil.
CA	<u>Cinnamon bark oil</u> – essential oil; anti-bacterial, anti-viral; anti-fungal; skin sensitizer; skin irritant; may cause light sensitivity; causescontact dermatitis; avoid if pregnant; see essential oils.

CA	<u>Cinnamon oil</u> - essential oil; skin and mucous membrane irritant; causes contact dermatitis; see cinnamon bark oil.
C	<u>Cinnamyl aldheyde</u> - see cinnamic aldehyde.
CA	<u>Cinoxate</u> - phototoxic chemical, causes photosensitivity, skin rashes.
†CA	<u>cis-9-octadecenoic acid</u> - see oleic acid.
C1	<u>Cistus ladaniferus</u> - see cistus oil.
C1	<u>Cistus oil</u> - essential oil; wound healing; use cautiously or avoid if pregnant; see essential oils.
C	<u>Citral</u> – inhibits tumor rejection and wound healing unless Vitamin A is present; causes contact dermatitis; sensitizer.
*CA	<u>Citratus</u> – see cymbopogon citratus.
*SA	<u>Citric acid</u> – skin and eye irrtant.
*S	<u>Citricidal</u> - see grapefruit seed extract.
C	<u>Citronella</u> – essential oil; may irritate sensitive skin; skin sensitizer if used frequently; inhalation of pure oil can increase heart rate; use cautiously or avoid if pregnant; see essential oils.
CA	<u>Citronellal hydrate</u> - see hydroxycitronella.
*S	<u>Citrus aurantifolia</u> – see lime oil.
*CA	<u>Citrus aurantium</u> – see orange oil.
S	<u>Citrus aurantium bigaradia</u> – see neroli oil.
*CA	<u>Citrus bergamia</u> – see bergamot oil.
CA	<u>Citrus lemon</u> – see lemon oil.
CA	<u>Citrus limomum</u> – see lemon oil.
S	<u>Citrus nobilus</u> – see tangerine oil.
S	<u>Citrus reticulata</u> – see mandarin oil.
C1	<u>Civet</u> – may irritate chemically sensitive individuals.
C1	<u>Clary sage oil</u> - essential oil; anti-septic; anti-fungal; astringent; infants and small children should avoid; avoid during/after alcohol consumption; use cautiously or avoid if pregnant.
CA	<u>Clove oil</u> - essential oil; skin irritant; causes contact dermatitis; frequent use may cause contact sensitization; use cautiously or avoid if pregnant; ban proposed for use in astringent products; see essential

oils.

XA   Coal tar – skin and eye irritant; phototoxic; carcinogen.

XA   Coal tar derivatives - skin irritant; may cause acne; sensitizer; carcinogen.

X   Cobalt - skin irritant; possible carcinogen.

X   Cobalt chloride – found in hair dyes; possible carcinogen.

†CA   Cocamide betaine - may cause formation of carcinogens in products containing nitrogen compounds.

†CA   Cocamide DEA - skin irritant, may cause formation of carcinogens in products containing nitrogen compounds; CIR panel says safe up to 10% concentrations in products that do not contain nitrosating agents; see DEA.

†CA   Cocamide diethanolamide – see cocamide DEA.

†CA   Cocamide diethanolamine – see cocamide DEA.

†CA   Cocamide MEA - skin irritant, may cause formation of carcinogens in products containing nitrogen compounds; see cocamide DEA, monoethanolamine.

†CA   Cocamide monoetanolamine - see cocamide MEA.

CA   Cocamide MIPA - skin irritant, may cause formation of carcinogens in products containing nitrogen compounds.

CA   Cocamide monoethanolamine - skin irritant, may cause formation of carcinogens in products containing nitrogen compounds; see monoethanolamine.

CA   Cocamide monoisopropanolamine – see cocamide MIPA.

†CA   Cocamidopropyl betaine – may contain a contaminant, amidoamine, which is a possible sensitizer; see coconut oil; CIR panel says safe with qualifications.

φCA   Cochineal extract – see carmine.

SA   Cocoa butter - may irritate skin, cause acne, allergic reactions.

33

CA Coco-betaine - see cocamidopropyl betaine.

CA Cocobetaine - see cocamidopropyl betaine.

SA Coconut oil - skin irritant.

†C Cocoyl sarcosine – mild cleanser; CIR panel says safe in "rinse-off" products, safe at 5% concentrations in "leave-on" products, insufficient data to determine safety in products which might be inhaled, may cause formation of carcinogens in products containing nitrogen compounds.

C Coffee extract – natural sunscreen; nervous system and adrenal gland stimulant; harmful in large amounts.

CA Colamine - see ethanolamine.

CA Collagen - allergic reactions common.

CA Colophony - skin irritant.

C Comfrey – herb; assists wound healing, may cause skin irritation; taken internally may cause liver damage.

C Comfrey extract – see comfrey.

*Cl Commiphora molmol – see myrrh oil.

*Cl Commiphora myrrha – see myrrh oil.

φS Copper powder – flammable.

S Coriander oil - essential oil; analgesic; anti-fungal; anti-bacterial; use sparingly; large doses may induce stupor; see essential oils.

S Coriandrum sativum – see coriander oil.

SA Corn oil - may cause acne.

CA Cornflower - herb, causes photosensitivity and allergy.

CA Cornflower distillate - phototoxic chemical, causes photosensitivity and allergy.

CA Cornflower extract - phototoxic chemical, causes photosensitivity and allergy; see extract.

CA Coumarin - may cause skin irritation, photosensitivity; toxic, carcinogenic if ingested.

X Crystalline silica – skin, eye and lung irritant; carcinogen; most harmful in dry powder form when inhaled.

S	Cucumber – herb; astringent.
S	Cucumis sativus - herb, astringent
CA	Cumarin - see coumarin.
C	Cumin oil - essential oil; herbal remedy; photosensitizer; antiviral; toxic if ingested; narcotic in large quantities.
C1	Cupressus sempervirens – see cypress oil.
X	Cyanide - poison.
C	Cyclohexamide - adversely affects skin; toxic if ingested.
X	Cyclopentasiloxane – not adequately tested; safety data not available.
*CA	Cymbopogon citratus – see lemongrass oil.
*CA	Cymbopogon flexuosis - see lemongrass oil.
S	Cymbopogon martini – see palmarosa oil.
C	Cymbopogon nardus – see citronella.
C1	Cypress oil - essential oil; astringent, insect repellant, deodorant; use cautiously or avoid if pregnant; see essential oils.
φXA	D&C Blue No. 4 – coal tar dye; potential carcinogen; see external use only, D&C Colors, coal tar.
XA	D&C Blue No. 4 Lake – may contain aluminum; see D&C Blue No. 4, aluminum powder.
φXA	D&C Brown No. 1 – mucous membrane and skin irritant; if absorbed into the body, can deplete oxygen and cause death; see external use only, D&C Colors.
φX	D&C Colors – colors considered safe by the FDA for drugs and cosmetics, but not for food; disregards permeability of the skin which allows these substances to be absorbed into the body; most of the colors are derived from coal tar and must be certified by the FDA not to contain more than 20ppm of lead and arsenic; certification does not address any harmful effects these colors may have on the body; most coal tar colors are potential carcinogens, may contain carcinogenic contaminants, and cause allergic reactions.

φXA   <u>D&C Green No. 5</u> – coal tar color; skin irritant; low toxicity; see D&C Colors; coal tar.

XA   <u>D&C Green No. 5 Lake</u> – may contain aluminum; see D&C Green No. 5, aluminum powder.

φXA   <u>D&C Green No. 6</u> – coal tar dye; skin irritant; potential carcinogen; see external use only, D&C Colors, coal tar.

XA   <u>D&C Green No. 6 Lake</u> – may contain aluminum; see D&C Green No. 6, aluminum powder.

φXA   <u>D&C Green No. 8</u> – pyrene color; potentially carcinogenic; see external use only, D&C Colors.

φXA   <u>D&C Orange No. 4</u> – monoazo dye; potential carcinogen; see external use only, D&C Colors.

XA   <u>D&C Orange No. 4 Lake</u> – may contain aluminum; see D&C Orange No. 4, aluminum powder.

φXA   <u>D&C Orange No. 5</u> – may cause cheilitis; carcinogen; see external use only, D&C Colors.

XA   <u>D&C Orange No. 5 Lake</u> – may contain aluminum; see D&C Orange No. 5, aluminum powder.

φXA   <u>D&C Orange No. 10</u> – coal tar color; possible photosensitizer, mutagen; see external use only, D&C Colors.

XA   <u>D&C Orange No. 10 Lake</u> – may contain aluminum; see D&C Orange No. 10, aluminum powder.

φXA   <u>D&C Orange No. 11</u> – coal tar color; see external use only, D&C Colors; coal tar.

XA   <u>D&C Orange No. 11 Lake</u> – may contain aluminum; see D&C Orange No. 11, aluminum powder.

X   <u>D&C Orange No. 17</u> – carcinogen; banned.

φXA   <u>D&C Red No. 6</u> – may cause acne; monoazo color; potential carcinogen; see D&C Colors, external use only.

XA   <u>D&C Red No. 6 Lake</u> – may contain aluminum; see D&C Red No. 6, aluminum powder.

φXA   <u>D&C Red No. 7</u> – may cause acne; monoazo color; potential carcinogen; see D&C Colors, external use only.

XA	D&C Red No. 7 Lake – may contain aluminum; see D&C Red No. 7, aluminum powder.
X	D&C Red No. 9 – carcinogen; banned.
φXA	D&C Red No. 17 – may cause acne; carcinogen; see external use only, D&C Colors, external use only.
XA	D&C Red No. 17 Lake – may contain aluminum; see D&C Red No. 17, aluminum powder.
X	D&C Red No. 19 – carcinogen; banned.
φXA	D&C Red No. 21 – coal tar color; may cause acne, cheilitis, photosensitivity; possible mutagen; see D&C Colors, external use only.
XA	D&C Red No. 21 Lake – may contain aluminum; see D&C Red No. 21, aluminum powder.
φXA	D&C Red No. 22 – coal tar color; potential carcinogen; may cause acne; see D&C Colors, external use only, coal tar.
XA	D&C Red No. 22 Lake – may contain aluminum; see D&C Red No. 22, aluminum powder.
φXA	D&C Red No. 27 – coal tar color; possible carcinogen; may cause acne, cheilitis; see D&C Colors, external use only, coal tar.
XA	D&C Red No. 27 Lake – may contain aluminum; see D&C Red No. 27, aluminum powder.
φXA	D&C Red No. 28 – coal tar color; possible carcinogen; may cause acne; see D&C Colors, external use only, coal tar.
XA	D&C Red No. 28 Lake – may contain aluminum; see D&C Red No. 28, aluminum powder.
φCA	D&C Red No. 30 – indigoid color; may cause acne; see D&C Colors, external use only.
CA	D&C Red No. 30 Lake – may contain aluminum; see D&C Red No. 30, aluminum powder.
φXA	D&C Red No. 31 – monoazo color; potential carcinogen; may cause acne; see external use only, D&C Colors.
XA	D&C Red No. 31 Lake – may contain aluminum; see D&C Red No. 31, aluminum powder.

φXA   D&C Red No. 33 – monoazo color; potential carcinogen; may cause acne; may contain carcinogenic impurities; see external use only, D&C Colors.

XA   D&C Red No. 33 Lake – may contain aluminum; may contain carcinogenic impurities; see D&C Red No. 33, aluminum powder.

φXA   D&C Red No. 34 – monoazo color; potential carcinogen; may cause acne; see external use only, D&C Colors.

XA   D&C Red No. 34 Lake – may contain aluminum; see D&C Red No. 34, aluminum powder.

φXA   D&C Red No. 36 – monoazo color; potential carcinogen; may cause acne, dermatitis; see external use only, D&C Colors.

XA   D&C Red No. 36 Lake – may contain aluminum; see D&C Red No. 36, aluminum powder.

φXA   D&C Violet No. 2 – coal tar dye; skin irritant; has caused tumors in rats; see external use only, D&C Colors, coal tar.

XA   D&C Violet No. 2 Lake – may contain aluminum; see D&C Violet No. 2, aluminum powder.

φXA   D&C Yellow No. 7 – coal tar color; mutagen; see external use only, D&C Colors, fluoresceins.

XA   D&C Yellow No. 7 Lake – may contain aluminum; see D&C Yellow No. 7, aluminum powder.

φXA   D&C Yellow No. 8 – coal tar color; potential carcinogen; see external use only, D&C Colors; coal tar.

XA   D&C Yellow No. 8 Lake – may contain aluminum; see D&C Yellow No. 8, aluminum powder.

φXA   D&C Yellow No. 10 – coal tar dye; skin irritant; potential carcinogen; see D&C Colors, external use only, coal tar.

XA   D&C Yellow No. 10 Lake – may contain aluminum; see D&C Yellow No. 10, aluminum powder.

φXA   D&C Yellow No. 11 – coal tar dye; skin irritant;

potential carcinogen; see external use only, D&C Colors, coal tar.

S   <u>Daucus carota</u> – see carrot oil.

C1   <u>Davana oil</u> – essential oil; use cautiously or avoid if pregnant.

†CA   <u>DEA</u> - mucous membrane, eye and skin irritant; absorbed through skin; carcinogen in mice; may cause formation of carcinogens with nitrogen containing compounds; may contain nitrosamine contaminants not listed on the label; CIR panel says safe up to 5% concentration in "rinse-off" products only.

CA   <u>DEA cetyl phosphate</u> - may cause formation of carcinogens; see DEA.

CA   <u>DEA dihydroxypalmityl phosphate</u> - may cause formation of carcinogens; see DEA.

CA   <u>DEA lauryl sulfate</u> - may cause formation of carcinogens; contains ammonium salts; see DEA, ammonia.

CA   <u>DEA methoxycinnamate</u> - phototoxic chemical, in sunlight may cause formation of carcinogenic nitrosamines; see DEA.

S   <u>Decyl oleate</u> - may cause acne.

C   <u>Denatured alcohol</u> – severe skin irritant; poisonous; inhalation may cause headaches, dizziness, difficulty breathing; ingestion may cause headaches, dizziness, blindness, coma, death.

S   <u>Deionized water</u>

C1   <u>Delphinensis</u> – see lavandin.

X   <u>Diamine</u> - skin and eye irritant; carcinogen.

X   <u>2,4-diaminoanisol</u> - carcinogen, mutagen, may cause genetic damage.

X   <u>2,5-diaminoanisol</u> - mutagen, may cause genetic damage.

X   <u>2,4-diaminoanisole sulfate</u> - carcinogen, mutagen, may cause genetic damage; contains ammonium salts, see ammonia.

X   <u>m-diaminobenzene</u> - see m-phenylenediamine.

XA   <u>1,2-diaminoethane</u> - see ethylenediamine.

X   <u>2,4-diaminotoluene</u> – causes dermatitis, sensitization; possible carcinogen; mutagen; may cause genetic damage; causes reproductive toxicity.

CA   <u>Diammonium dithiodiglycolate</u> - skin irritant.

†C   <u>Diazolidinyl urea</u> - preservative; skin irritant; may release formaldehyde; CIR panel says safe up to .5% concentration; see formaldehyde.

CA   <u>Dibromocyanobutane</u> - skin irritant; preservative.

C   <u>1,2-dibromo-2,4-dicyanobutane</u> - causes eczema.

X   <u>Dichlorobenzyl alcohol</u> – not tested for safety; see benzyl alcohol.

X   <u>1,2-dichloroethane</u> – carcinogen.

XA   <u>Dichlorophen</u> - toxic; skin and eye irritant; may cause diarrhea and cramps; potent allergen.

†CA   <u>Diethanolamine</u> - see DEA.

C   <u>Diethyl maleate</u> – causes contact dermatitis.

X   <u>1,4-diethylene dioxide</u> - see 1,4-dioxane.

X   <u>Diethylene ether</u> - see 1,4-dioxane.

X   <u>Diethylene glycol</u> – toxic; absorbs through skin; hazardous if used on large areas of the body; ingestion can be fatal.

X   <u>Diethylene oxide</u> - see 1,4-dioxane.

X   <u>Diethylnitrosamine</u> – carcinogen.

C   <u>Digalloyl trioleate</u> - phototoxic chemical, causes photosensitivity.

C   <u>5,7-dihydroxy-4-methyl coumarin</u> - sensitizes skin.

φCA   <u>Dihydroxyacetone</u> – skin irritant; has caused death when large doses injected into rats; see external use only.

C   <u>5,7-dihydroxycoumarin</u> - sensitizes skin.

X   <u>Diisopropanolnitrosamine</u> – carcinogen; contains ammonium salts, see ammonia.

C   <u>Dimethicon</u> - has caused mutations and tumors in lab animals.

†CA   <u>Dimethicone</u> - use on skin may cause internal problems; low toxicity; CIR says safe as used in cosmetics; see silica.

CA   Dimethicone copolyol - see dimethicone.
CA   3,7-dimethyl-7-hydroxyoctenal - see hydroxycitronella.
CA   3,7-dimethyl-1,6-octadien-3-ol - see linalool.
CA   Dimethyl lauramine - may cause formation of carcinogens; insufficient data to support safety according to CIR panel.
CA   Dimethyl stearamine - may cause formation of carcinogens; insufficient data to support safety according to CIR panel.
X   Dimethylamine – severe eye, skin, mucous membrane irritant; absorbed through skin; may be fatal if inhaled; see ammonia.
X   Dimethylnitrosamine - carcinogen; easily absorbed through skin; contains ammonium salt, see ammonia.
X   Dioctyl phthalate – eye, skin and mucous membrane irritant; carcinogen; central nervous system depressant.
*X   Dioctyl sodium sulfosuccinate – see sodiumsulfosuccinate.
*X   Dioctyl sulfosuccinate sodium – see sodiumsulfosuccinate.
C   Dioctyl sebacate – skin and eye irritant; inhalation may cause nausea, respiratory tract irritation; flammable.
X   Dioxane - industrial poison; carcinogen.
X   1,4-dioxane - carcinogen; found in 40% of cosmetics; absorbed through skin; toxic if inhaled; may be removed during processing by vacuum stripping, but product labels do not give adequate information to determine if the product is contaminated.
C   Dioxybenzone - see benzophenone.
X   Dioxyethylene ether - see 1,4-dioxane.
†C   Diphenylketone – see benzophenone.
X   Direct black 38 – carcinogen.
X   Direct blue 6 – carcinogen.
X   Diresorcinolphthalein - see fluoresceins.
CA   Disodium EDTA - may cause formation of

41

carcinogens in products containing nitrogen compounds; mucous membrane, eye and skin irritant; may cause asthma, kidney damage.

φCA   Disodium EDTA-copper – approved for shampoo only; see disodium EDTA

C   Disodium laureth sulfosuccinate - may contain toxic byproducts; see ethoxylated alcohols.

C   Disodium oleamido PEG - may contain toxic byproducts; see ethoxylated alcohols.

S   Disodium phosphate – skin and eye irritant.

CA   Disodium salt – see disodium EDTA.

X   DMD hydantoin - preservative; may contain formaldehyde.

†X   DMDM hydantoin - may cause dermatitis; may contain formaldehyde; hydantoin has caused cancer in rats; see formaldehyde.

S   1-dodecanol - see lauryl alcohol.

S   Dodecyl alcohol - see lauryl alcohol.

XA   p-dohydroxybenzene - see hydroquinone.

CA   Dowicil - preservative; may cause allergic reactions.

CA   Dyes – soluble colors, usually petroleum based; see coal tar derivatives, hair dyes.

S   Echinacea – herb; heals damaged skin; immune system stimulant.

S   Echinacea angustifolia – see echinacea.

CA   EDTA - see disodium EDTA.

S   Elastin – a protein in the skin; elastin in cosmetics is derived from animals and cannot changed the elasticity of human skin; it moisturizes the skin.

S   Elemi oil – essential oil; antiseptic; aids allergic rashes, chapped skin.

X   Epoxyethane - see ethylene oxide.

C1   Equisetum arvense – see horse tail.

XA   Erythrosine Potassium - see coal tar derivatives.

XA   Erythrosine Sodium - see coal tar derivatives.

X   Essence of mirabane - see nitrobenzene.

C   Essence of Niobe - see ethyl benzoate.

C   Essential oils – properly extracted for highest purity

and used knowledgeably, essential oils have great therapeutic benefit; if solvent or heat extracted, they are highly refined and lose beneficial properties; toxic solvent extraction contaminants may remain in the finished product.

XA   1,2-ethanediol - see ethylene glycol.

C   Ethanol - see ethyl alcohol.

CA   Ethanolamine – severe nose, throat, eye and skin irritant; absorbed through skin; central nervous system depressant; may cause kidney, liver damage; may cause formation of carcinogens in products containing nitrogen compounds; mutagen.

CA   Ethanolamines – see ethanolamine.

C   Ether - skin irritant; may cause central nervous system depression if inhaled or ingested.

C   Ethers - skin irritant; may cause central nervous system depression if inhaled or ingested.

X   Ethoxyethanol - CIR panel determined this ingredient to be unsafe.

X   Ethoxyethanol acetate - CIR panel determined this ingredient to be unsafe.

CA   2-ethoxyethyl-p-methoxy cinnamate - phototoxic chemical, causes photosensitivity, skin rashes.

C   Ethoxylated alcohols – may contain carcinogenic contaminant, 1,4-dioxane, which is rapidly absorbed through the skin; may be removed during processing by vacuum stripping, but product labels do not give adequate information to determine if the product is contaminated.

CA   Ethoxylated lanolins - skin irritant; may cause acne; may contain harmful amounts of toxic byproducts.

†C   Ethyl acetate – skin irritant; may cause liver, kidney damage, central nervous system depression.

C   Ethyl alcohol - drying to skin and hair; may cause contact dermatitis; eye irritant; carcinogen and mutagen if swallowed.

C   Ethyl benzenecarboxylate - see ethyl benzoate.

C   Ethyl benzoate - eye and skin irritant; toxic if

swallow large amounts.

†S   <u>Ethyl ester of PVM/MA copolymer</u> – toxic if inhaled; CIR panel says safe as used in cosmetics.

CA   <u>Ethyl-p-aminobenzoate</u> - may cause contact dermatitis, has caused oxygen loss in the blood of babies, central nervous system irritability in adults.

CA   <u>Ethyl-p-hydroxybenzoate</u> - preservative; skin irritant; strong allergen; toxic.

XA   <u>Ethylene alcohol</u> - see ethylene glycol.

XA   <u>Ethylene glycol</u> - can cause contact dermatitis; may cause kidney, liver, respiratory problems, death; toxic if inhaled; mutagen; neurotoxin; hazardous if used on large areas of the body; can be fatal if ingested.

X   <u>Ethylene oxide</u> - skin and eye irritant; may cause kidney damage; harmful if swallowed; carcinogen; may cause inheritable genetic damage.

XA   <u>Ethylenediamine</u> - skin and eye irritant; sensitizer; may cause asthma; toxic if inhaled or absorbed through skin.

CA   <u>Ethylenediaminetetraacetic acid</u> – see disodium EDTA.

CA   <u>Ethylparaben</u> - see ethyl-p-hydroxybenzoate.

C   <u>Eucalyptus citriodora</u> – see eucalyptus oil (lemon scented).

S   <u>Eucalyptus globulus</u> - essential oil, antibacterial, anti-inflammatory, insect repellant.

S   <u>Eucalyptus oil</u> - essential oil; antibacterial, anti-inflammatory, insect repellant; toxic if taken internally.

C   <u>Eucalyptus oil (lemon scented)</u> – essential oil; frequent use may cause contact sensitization; toxic if taken internally.

CA   <u>Eugenia caryophyllus</u> – see clove oil.

*CA   <u>Eugenol</u> – skin irritant; causes contact dermatitis; mutagen; toxic if swallowed.

φC   <u>External use only</u> – the FDA has approved, as safe, some colorants "for external use only" disregarding the fact that substances put on the skin can be absorbed into the body. If these substances are harmful when ingested, they will still be harmful when absorbed into the body.

φX Ext. D&C Colors - colors considered safe by the FDA for drugs and cosmetics used externally on the skin, but not on the mucous membranes or for food; disregards permeability of the skin which allows these substances to be absorbed into the body; most of the colors are derived from coal tar and must be certified by the FDA not to contain more than 20ppm of lead and arsenic; certification does not address any harmful effects these colors may have on the body; most coal tar colors are potential carcinogens, may contain carcinogenic contaminants and cause allergic reactions.

φXA Ext. D&C Violet No. 2 – coal tar color; see D&C Violet No. 2; see external use only, Ext. D&C Colors; coal tar.

φXA Ext. D&C Yellow No. 7 – coal tar color; skin irritant; potential carcinogen; see external use only, Ext. D&C Colors; coal tar.

XA Ext. D&C Yellow No. 7 Lake – may contain aluminum; see Ext. D&C Yellow No. 7, aluminum powder.

C Extract – extraction may be by cold or hot hydraulic pressing or by organic solvents; solvent extraction requires the solvent to be refined out and may leave toxic contaminant residue in the extract; hot pressing and solvent extraction cause loss of beneficial substances and are highly refined; only cold pressing preserves beneficial ingredients.

S Extract of aloe vera – see aloe, extract.

S Extract of balm mint – no known toxicity; see extract.

C1 Extract of burdock – see burdock, extract.

S Extract of calendula - see calendula, extract.

SA Extract of chamomile - see chamomile, extract.

S	<u>Extract of coltsfoot</u> – large doses may cause liver damage; see extract.
C	<u>Extract of comfrey</u> - see comfrey, extract.
S	<u>Extract of cucumber</u> - see extract.
S	<u>Extract of grapefruit</u> - see extract
C1	<u>Extract of horsetail</u> - see horsetail, extract.
C1A	<u>Extract of hypericum</u> - see hypericum perforatum, extract.
SA	<u>Extract of ivy</u> - see ivy extract, extract.
SA	<u>Extract of matricaria</u> - see chamomile, extract.
S	<u>Extract of orchid</u> - see extract.
C1	<u>Extract of sambucus</u> – diuretic; avoid if pregnant; only sambucus nigra is safe; sambucus ebulus and sambucus racemosa are toxic; see extract.
S	<u>Extract of stinging nettle</u> - see nettle, extract.
S	<u>Extract of valerian</u> - see valerian oil, extract.
S	<u>Extract of yarrow</u> - see yarrow oil, extract.
S	<u>Fatty acids</u> - necessary for good health; a German study found carcinogenic contaminants.
S	<u>Fatty acid esters</u> – no known toxicity.
CA	<u>Fatty alcohols</u> - may cause allergic reaction, skin irritation; low toxicity.
C	<u>Fatty amine oxides</u> - may be contaminated with carcinogens.
φXA	<u>FD&C Blue No. 1</u> – coal tar dye; carcinogen; see FD&C Colors, coal tar.
XA	<u>FD&C Blue No. 1 Lake</u> - coal tar dye; carcinogen; may contain aluminum; see FD&C Colors, aluminum powder.
XA	<u>FD&C Blue No. 2</u> - coal tar dye; potential carcinogen; see FD&C Colors; coal tar.
XA	<u>FD&C Blue No. 2 Lake</u> - coal tar dye; potential carcinogen; may contain aluminum; see FD&C Colors, aluminum powder.
φX	<u>FD&C Colors</u> – colors considered safe by the FDA for use in food, drugs and cosmetics; most of the colors are derived from coal tar and must be certified by the FDA not to contain more than 10ppm of lead

and arsenic; certification does not address any harmful effects these colors may have on the body; most coal tar colors are potential carcinogens, may contain carcinogenic contaminants, and cause allergic reactions.

φXA FD&C Green No. 3 – carcinogen; see FD&C Colors.

XA FD&C Green No. 3 Lake – may contain aluminum; see FD&C Green No. 3, aluminum powder.

XA FD&C Red No. 3 - carcinogen, color derived from coal tar; banned for cosmetics and drugs used externally; still approved for use in foods and drugs taken internally; see FD&C Colors, coal tar.

φXA FD&C Red No. 4 – coal tar dye; causes atrophied adrenal glands and bladder polyps in animals, banned in food and drugs, but allowed in cosmetics; see external use only, FD&C Colors, coal tar.

XA FD&C Red No. 4 Lake – may contain aluminum; see FD&C Red No. 4, aluminum powder.

φXA FD&C Red No. 40 – monoazo color; suspected carcinogen; may be contaminated with carcinogens; see FD&C Colors.

φXA FD&C Red No. 40 Aluminum Lake – may be contaminated with a carcinogen; see FD&C Colors, aluminum powder.

φXA FD&C Yellow No. 5 – coal tar dye; potential carcinogen; may contain carcinogenic contaminants; aspirin sensitive individuals may develop life-threatening symptoms; see FD&C Colors.

XA FD&C Yellow No. 5 Lake – may contain aluminum; see FD&C Yellow No. 5, aluminum powder.

φXA FD&C Yellow No. 6 – coal tar dye; potential carcinogen; may contain carcinogenic contaminants; see FD&C Colors, coal tar.

XA FD&C Yellow No. 6 Lake – may contain aluminum; see FD&C Yellow No. 6, aluminum powder.

*CA Fennel oil – essential oil; skin irritant; antiseptic; frequent use may cause contact sentization; mutagen;

toxic if swallow large amounts; avoid if kidney problems; use cautiously or avoid if pregnant or epileptic; see essential oils.

φC   <u>Ferric ammonium ferrocyanide</u> – see external use only.

φC   <u>Ferric ferrocyanide</u> – see external use only.

S   <u>Ferula gummose</u> – see galbanum.

S   <u>Fir oil</u> - essential oil; irritant to sensitive skin.

S   <u>Flavonoids</u> – herbs; tone skin; strengthen capillaries.

SA   <u>Flaxseed oil</u> - see linseed oil.

X   <u>Fluoranthene</u> – mutagen; not adequately tested for carcinogenic effects.

X   <u>Fluoresceins</u> - may damage DNA and cause mutations, tumors or neoplasms.

X   <u>Fluoride</u> – skin, eye, nose, throat irritant; poison; causes premature aging, weakening of the immune system, mottling of the teeth, anemia, joint stiffness, calcified ligaments, genetic damage.

*CA   <u>Foeniculum vulgare</u> – see fennel oil.

†XA   <u>Formaldehyde</u> - carcinogen, mutagen; neurotoxin; sensitizer; eye and skin irritant; poison if swallowed; CIR panel says safe up to .2% free formaldehyde, not safe in aerosol products; banned in Japan and Sweden.

XA   <u>Formalin</u> - see formaldehyde.

XA   <u>Formic aldehyde</u> - see formaldehyde.

XA   <u>Formol</u> - see formaldehyde.

CA   <u>Fragrance</u> - may irritate skin; may cause cheilitis; manufacturers are not required to disclose chemicals used for fragrance; some hazardous chemicals found in fragrance include benzyl chloride, ethyl alcohol, methylene chloride, methyl ethyl ketone, methyl isobutyl ketone and toluene; may contain carcinogens.

S   <u>Frankincense oil</u> - essential oil; antiseptic; antidepressant; immune-stimulant; see essential oils.

X   <u>Furocoumarines</u> - phototoxic chemical; may damage DNA and cause mutations, tumors or neoplasms.

X   Furocoumarin-plus-UVA - phototoxic chemical; may damage DNA and cause mutations, tumors or neoplasms.

S   Galbanum – essential oil; antiseptic; anti-inflammatory; potential irritant for the chemically sensitive; see essential oils.

S   Garlic – herb; antibacterial; fresh juice may cause burns.

S   Garlic oil – see garlic.

SA   Geraniol - occurs naturally in fruits, herbs and essential oils; may irritate skin.

SA   Geranium oil - essential oil; astringent; antiseptic; insect repellant; may irritate skin; frequent use may cause contact sensitization; harmful if ingested.

S   Ginger oil - essential oil; antiseptic; may cause photosensitivity; frequent use may cause contact sensitization.

S   Ginseng – herb; demulcent; stimulant; may increase cell life; may cause vaginal bleeding.

X   Glutamic acid – skin, eye, respiratory and digestive irritant; mutagen, may cause birth defects; harmful if absorbed through skin, swallowed or inhaled; suspected carcinogen; not adequately tested.

*S   Glycerin - see glycerol

*S   Glycerine - see glycerol

*S   Glycerol – in concentrated from, may irritate eyes, skin and mucous membranes; harmful if absorbed through skin; nontoxic as used; may be derived from animal and vegetable fats and oils or produced synthetically from petroleum; safety claims not proven in diaper-rash, poison ivy, oak and sumac products.

SA   Glycerol monolaurate – skin irritant.

SA   Glycerol monostearate - eye irritant.

SA   Glyceryl monolaurate – skin irritant.

SA   Glyceryl monostearate – eye irritant.

†SA   Glyceryl oleate - CIR panel says safe as used up to 5% concentration.

CA   <u>Glyceryl PABA</u> - may cause photosensitivity, skin irritation.

X   <u>Glyceryl ricinoleate</u> - insufficient data to support safety according to CIR panel; not adequately tested.

SA   <u>Glyceryl stearate</u> – see glyceryl monostearate.

†CA   <u>Glyceryl thioglycolate</u> - skin irritant in permanent solutions; potential sensitizer; CIR panel says this is a potential sensitizer, but infrequent use can be safe.

*S   <u>Glycyl alcohol</u> - see glycerol.

XA   <u>Glycol</u> – hazardous when used on large areas of the body; see ethylene glycol.

CA   <u>Glycol distearate</u> - may irritate eyes, skin and mucous membranes; may be contaminated with ethylene glycol; see ethylene glycol.

†C   <u>Glycolic acid</u> – see alpha hydroxy acids.

C1   <u>Goldenseal extract</u> – natural antibiotic; immune system stimulant; aids digestion; healing to skin and mucous membranes; may increase blood pressure, stimulate uterus; avoid if pregnant or hypertensive; toxic in large amounts.

C1   <u>Gotu kola</u> – herb; anti-wrinkle; anti-aging properties; avoid if pregnant or lactating.

C   <u>Grain alcohol</u> - see ethyl alcohol.

*S   <u>Graprfruit seed extract</u> – preservative; non-toxic; effective in clearing up eczema, rashes, lip blisters, herpes, skin fungi and other skin irritation.

S   <u>Grapeseed oil</u> – essential oil carrier; astringent.

φXA   <u>Green No. 3</u> – carcinogen; see FD&C Green No. 3.

φC   <u>Guaiazulene</u> - not adequately tested; CIR panel states insufficient data to support safety; see external use only.

φS   <u>Guanine</u>

XA   <u>Guar hydroxypropyltrimonium chloride</u> – see quarternary ammonium compounds.

X   <u>Hair dyes</u> – cause cancer, but do not require a warning on the label; increase risk of multiple myeloma, Hodgkin's disease, non-Hodgkin's lymphoma and possibly breast cancer.

CA   Hamamelis virginiana – see witch hazel.

X   HC Blue No. 1 – carcinogen; CIR panel determined this ingredient to be unsafe.

S   Helichrysum – essential oil; antioxidant; sunscreen; see essential oils.

S   Helichrysum italicum – see helichrysum.

φSA   Henna – skin irritant; avoid use near eyes; limited to hair dyes.

X   Hexachlorophene – extremely toxic; use prohibited unless physician prescribes.

†C   Hexadecanoic acid - see palmitic acid.

†C   2,4-hexadienoic acid – see sorbic acid.

†CA   Hexamethylenetetramine - see methenamine.

C   Hexamidine diisethionate - skin irritant; petroleum based; many petroleum products are carcinogens.

XA   Hexylene glycol - eye, skin, mucous membrane irritant; toxic if inhaled or ingested; hazardous if used on large areas of the body.

SA   Heliotrope oil – see violet oil.

†CA   HMTA - see methenamine.

CA   Homosalate – coal tar derivative; may cause allergic reaction.

CA   Homomenthyl salicylate - see salicylic acid.

S   Hops – herb; antimicrobial; antiaging; may cause dermatitis.

S   Horse chestnut - herb, anti-inflammatory, for sensitive skin, capillary fragility.

C1   Horsetail – herb; avoid if pregnant; excess may cause birth defects.

S   Humulus lupulus – see hops.

C   Hydantoins - skin irritant; has caused cancer in rats.

X   Hydrazine - skin and eye irritant; carcinogen.

C1   Hydrocotyle asiatica – see gotu kola.

*C   Hydrogen peroxide - toxic if inhaled or large amounts ingested; mutagen; skin irritant undiluted; 3% solution considered safe as antiseptic, gargle; not proven safe for poison ivy, poison oak, poison sumac.

CA   Hydrogenated vegetable oil – consumption is associated with heart disease, breast and colon cancer, atherosclerosis, elevated cholesterol.

C   Hydrolyzed – may contain hidden MSG; see MSG.

C   Hydrolyzed whole wheat protein – may contain hidden MSG; see msg.

XA   Hydroquinol - see hydroquinone.

†XA   Hydroquinone - may cause severe skin damage; toxic if inhaled or ingested; ingesting less than 1 ounce may be fatal; has caused cancer in mice; CIR panel says safe at .1% concentrations or less for brief, "rinse-off" use only; see external use only.

CA   Hydroxy citronellal – skin and eye irritant; may cause psoriasis, contact dermatitis; harmful if swallowed.

X   p-hydroxyanisole - CIR panel determined this ingredient to be unsafe.

C   Hydroxybenzoic acids – see salicylic acid.

CA   Hydroxycitronella – see hydroxy citronellal.

CA   Hydroxycoumarins - skin irritant; may cause photosensitivity; coumarin is a carcinogen and banned in food.

CA   2-hydroxyethylamine - see ethanolamine.

SA   Hydroxyethylcellulose

C   2-hydroxy-4-methoxybenzophenone - can cause serious contact dermatitis.

C   Hydroxymethylcellulose – see carboxymethyl cellulose.

CA   2-hydroxypropyl amine – see monoisopropanolamine.

C   Hydroxypropyl aminobenzoate - may cause formation of carcinogens in products containing nitrogen compounds.

†S   Hydroxypropyl cellulose - slight skin and eye irritant.

†S   Hydroxy propylmethyl cellulose - skin and eye irritant.

C1A   Hypericum perforatum – herb; essential oil: anti-inflammatory; antibiotic; astringent; skin irritant; causes photosensitivity; avoid if pregnant.

C1A   <u>Hypericum perforatum extract</u> – herb; essential oil: anti-inflammatory; antibiotic; astringent; skin irritant; causes photosensitivity; avoid if pregnant; insufficient data to support safety according to CIR panel.

C1A   <u>Hypericum perforatum oil</u> – herb; essential oil: anti-inflammatory; antibiotic; astringent; skin irritant; causes photosensitivity; avoid if pregnant; insufficient data to support safety according to CIR panel.

C   <u>Hyssop oil</u> - essential oil; astringent; antiseptic; contains pinocamphone which may be toxic; avoid if pregnant, epileptic or high blood pressure.

C   <u>Hyssopus officinalis</u> - see hyssop oil.

†C   <u>Imidazolidinyl urea</u> - preservative; strong irritant; causes contact deramtitis; may contain formaldehyde; see formaldehyde.

S   <u>Indian Cress</u> - herb, antibacterial, antifungal

*S   <u>Inositol</u> - a B vitamin; see nutrient additives.

CA   <u>Iodine</u> – skin and eye irritant; may cause asthma or anaphylactic shock in susceptible individuals.

φS   <u>Iron oxides</u> – skin and eye irritant; lung irritant if inhaled, may cause siderosis.

†C   <u>Isobutane</u> – propellant; flammable; neurotoxin.

C   <u>Isoceteth-n</u> - may contain toxic byproducts; see ethoxylated alcohols.

SA   <u>Isocetyl laurate</u> - see isocetyl stearate.

SA   <u>Isocetyl stearate</u> - skin irritant; may cause acne.

X   <u>Isoeugenol</u> – strong skin irritant; mutagen; toxic if swallowed.

C   <u>Isolaureth-n</u> - may contain toxic byproducts; see ethoxylated alcohols.

†C   <u>Isopentane</u> – petroleum derivative; skin irritant; flammable; narcotic in large amounts.

†CA   <u>Isopropanolamine</u> – CIR panel says safe with qualifications; see monoisopropanloamine.

C   <u>4-isopropyl-dibenzoylmethane</u> - can cause contact dermatitis.

CA   <u>Isopropyl-hydroxypalmityl-ether</u> - may cause allergic reactions.

†S   <u>Isopropyl isostearate</u> - may cause acne.

†XA   <u>Isopropyl myristate</u> - may cause acne, irritate skin; may increase absorption of toxic/carcinogenic contaminants by more than 200 times.

†SA   <u>Isopropyl palmitate</u> - may irritate skin, cause acne.

C   <u>Isopsoralen</u> - causes phototoxicity.

†C   <u>Isostearamide DEA</u> - may cause formation of carcinogens in products containing nitrogen compounds; CIR panel says safe up to 40 percent concentration; see DEA.

†C   <u>Isostearamide MEA</u> – see isostearamide DEA.

C   <u>Isosteareth -20</u> - may contain toxic byproducts; see ethoxylated alcohols.

C   <u>Isosteareth -n</u> - may contain toxic byproducts; see ethoxylated alcohols.

†C   <u>Isostearic acid</u> – skin, eye and mucous membrane irritant; potential sensitizer; not adequately tested.

†S   <u>Isostearyl neopentanoate</u> - may cause acne.

CA   <u>Isothiazolinones</u> - preservative; may irritate skin, cause allergic reaction, mostly in those with nickel allergies; mutagen.

S   <u>Ispaghul extract</u> – see plantago.

SA   <u>Ivy extract</u> - skin irritant; may cause dermatitis; toxic if taken internally.

S   <u>Jasmine</u> – see essential oils.

S   <u>Jasmine absolute</u> - essential oil; antiseptic; anti-inflammatory; antibacterial; see essential oils.

S   <u>Jasminum officinale</u> – see jasmine absolute.

†S A   <u>Jojoba oil</u> – healing to skin, natural sunscreen if cold pressed; heat pressed or solvent extracted is highly refined and loses healing properties.

S   <u>Juniper oil</u> - essential oil; antibacterial; anti-inflammatory; astringent; detoxifier; see essential oils.

S   <u>Juniperus communis</u> – see juniper oil.

CA   <u>Kathon CG</u> – sensitizer; skin and eye irritant;

mutagen; toxic.

S   Keratin protein – a component of skin, nails and hair.

X   Kohl - causes lead poisoning.

†C   Lactic acid – see alpha hydroxy acids.

†CA   Lanolin - skin irritant; sensitizer; may cause cheilitis; safety and effectiveness not shown for poison oak, ivy and sumac products; may be contaminated with carcinogenic and neurotoxic pesticides which may be absorbed through the skin into the bloodstream; should be avoided by nursing mothers, infants and children.

CA   Lanolin alcohol - may cause acne; less irritating than lanolin; may be contaminated with carcinogenic and neurotoxic pesticides; should be avoided by nursing mothers and infants and children.

†CA   Lanolin oil – may be less irritating to skin than lanolin; may be contaminated with carcinogenic and neurotoxic pesticides; should be avoided by nursing mothers and infants and children.

†C   Lauramide DEA - may cause formation of carcinogens in products containing nitrogen compounds; CIR panel says safe up to 10% concentrations in products that do not contain nitrosating agents; see DEA.

CA   Lauramidopropyl dimethylamine - skin, mucous membrane irritant.

*CA   Laurel oil – essential oil; frequent use may cause contact sensitization; skin irritant; toxic if ingested; use cautiously or avoid if pregnant; see essential oils.

†C   Laureth-1, -23 - may contain toxic byproducts; see ethoxylated alcohols.

*CA   Laurus nobilis – see laurel oil.

†C   Lauroyl sarcosine – CIR panel says safe in "rinse-off" products, safe at 5% concentrations in "leave-on" products, insufficient data to determine safety in products which might be inhaled, may cause formation of carcinogens in products containing nitrogen compounds.

S   <u>Lauryl alcohol</u> - may cause acne, irritate skin.

C1   <u>Lavandin</u> – essential; antiseptic; anti-inflammatory; avoid if pregnant; use cautiously or avoid if epileptic; see lavender oil.

C1   <u>Lavandula Delphinensis</u> – see lavandin.

C1   <u>Lavandula Fragrans</u> – see lavandin.

*SA   <u>Lavandula officinalis</u> – see lavender oil.

*SA   <u>Lavender oil</u> - essential oil; antiseptic; anti-inflammatory; may cause photosensitivity; skin irritant: toxic if ingested in large amounts.

*SA   <u>Lavendula officinalis</u> - see lavender oil.

φX   <u>Lead acetate</u> – absorption through skin may cause lead poisoning; carcinogen; limited to hair dyes.

†C   <u>Lecithin</u> – CIR says safe in "rinse-off" products, safe in "leave-on" products up to 15% concentration, insufficient data to determine safety where ingredients might be inhaled, may cause formation of carcinogens in products containing nitrogen compounds.

SA   <u>Lemon</u> – see lemon juice.

S   <u>Lemon balm</u> – see melissa oil.

S   <u>Lemon balm oil</u> – see melissa oil.

CA   <u>Lemon essence</u> - see lemon oil.

CA   <u>Lemon extract</u> - see lemon oil.

SA   <u>Lemon juice</u> – may cause photosensitivity; may irritate the skin.

CA   <u>Lemon oil</u> - essential oil from lemon peel; may cause phototoxicity; antiseptic; antibacterial; anti-aging properties; may cause contact dermatitis; suspected co-carcinogen; see essential oils.

SA   <u>Lemon peel</u>

CA   <u>Lemon peel oil</u> – see lemon oil.

*CA   <u>Lemongrass oil</u> - essential oil; skin irritant; antibacterial; antifungal; insect repellant; mildly toxic if swallow large amounts; has caused death when ingested; topical safety unknown; use small amounts; avoid with glaucoma; caution with sensitive or damaged skin and prostatic hyperplasia; avoid with children.

*S <u>Lime essence</u> – see lime oil.

*SA <u>Lime juice</u> – see lemon juice.

*S <u>Lime oil</u> – essential oil; antiseptic; anti-bacterial; anti-viral; causes photosensitivity; see essential oils.

C <u>d-limonene</u> – sensitizer; skin and eye irritant; inadequate evidence of carcinogenity; teratogen; neurotoxin.

SA <u>Linalol</u> - see linalool.

SA <u>Linalool</u> - skin irritant.

†C <u>Lineoleamide DEA</u> - can cause formation of carcinogens in products containing nitrogen compounds; CIR panel says safe, but should not be used in products with nitrosating agents; see DEA.

C <u>Linoleamidopropyl ethydimonium ethosulfate</u> - may cause formation of carcinogens in products containing nitrogen compounds; skin and mucous membrane irritant; contains ammonium salts, see ammonia.

SA <u>Linseed oil</u> - may cause acne.

C <u>Magnesium laureth sulfate</u> - may contain toxic byproducts; contains ammonium salts; see ammonia, ethoxylated alcohols.

C <u>Magnesium oleth sulfate</u> - may contain toxic byproducts; contains ammonium salts; see ammonia, ethoxylated alcohols.

SA <u>Maize oil</u> - see corn oil.

†C <u>Malic acid</u> – CIR panel says safe as pH adjusters only, insufficient data to determine safety for any other use.

S <u>Mallow</u> – herb; antiallergenic; anti-inflammatory; for sensitive skin.

S <u>Malva sylvestries</u> – see mallow.

S <u>Mandarin oil</u> – essential oil; antiseptic; gentle; may be used for children and during pregnancy; causes photosensitivity.

φS <u>Manganese violet</u> – toxic if inhaled.

S <u>Marigold</u> – herb; soothes inflammation; may cause

dermatitis.

S   <u>Marigold oil</u> – may cause photosensitivity; see marigold, oils.

C1   <u>Marjoram oil</u> – essential oil; antiseptic; anti-bacterial; use cautiously or avoid if pregnant; see essential oils.

S   <u>Marsh mallow</u> – herb; may heal eczema, dermatitis.

SA   <u>Matricaria chamomilla</u> – see chamomile.

CA   <u>MEA</u> - see monoethanolamine.

C1   <u>Meadowsweet oil</u> - essential oil; avoid if aspirin sensitive, pregnant; do not give to children with chicken-pox, colds, flu.

S   <u>Melaleuca alternifolia</u> - essential oil; antiseptic; anti-bacterial; anti-fungal; anti-viral; frequent use may cause contact sensitization; see essential oils.

S   <u>Melaleuca ericifolia</u> – see rosalina.

C   <u>Melaleuca leucadendron</u> – see cajaput oil.

S   <u>Melaleuca quinquenervia</u> - see melaleuca alternifolia.

S   <u>Melaleuca viridiflora</u> - essential oil; see melaleuca alternifolia.

S   <u>Melissa balm oil</u> – see melissa oil.

S   <u>Melissa oil</u> - essential oil; insect repellant; antibacterial; may interfere with thyroid hormones; often distilled with other oils; may not be pure; external use only; see essential oils.

S   <u>Melissa officinalis</u> – see melissa oil.

C1A   <u>Mentha piperita</u> – see peppermint oil.

C1   <u>Mentha spicata</u> – see spearmint oil.

C   <u>Menthol</u> – eye irritant; moderately toxic if swallowed in large amounts; local anesthetic; may cause changes in the mucous membranes if used for long periods in concentrations greater than 3%; not shown safe and effective in over-the-counter products.

X   <u>Mercuric ammonium chloride</u> – poison; mercury compounds are prohibited except as preservatives in eye cosmetics; see ammonia.

X   <u>Mercuric chloride</u> – poison; mercury compounds are prohibited except as preservatives in eye cosmetics.

X   <u>Mercuric chloride ammoniated</u> - toxic; skin irritant;

mercury compounds are prohibited except as preservatives in eye cosmetics; see ammonia.

XA   Methanal - see formaldehyde.

†C   Methaninie - causes dermatitis; skin irritant; causes birth defects in rats when ingested; releases formaldehyde.

X   Methanol - see methyl alcohol.

†CA   Methenamine - causes skin rashes; flammable.

X   Methenammonium chloride – see ammonia.

X   Methoxsalen - phototoxic chemical, causes photosensitivity, may damage DNA and cause mutations, tumors or neoplasms; carcinogen.

X   2-methoxyaniline – carcinogen.

X   4-methoxyaniline – carcinogen.

X   4-methoxy-3-phenylenediamine – carcinogen.

X   4-methoxy-m-phenylenediamine – carcinogen; CIR panel determined this ingredient to be unsafe.

X   4-methoxy-m-phenylenediamine HCl – CIR panel determined this ingredient to be unsafe.

X   4-methoxy-m-phenylenediamine sulfate – CIR panel determined this ingredient to be unsafe; contains ammonium salts, see ammonia.

X   5-methoxypsoralen - phototoxic chemical, may damage DNA and cause mutations, tumors or neoplasms; probable carcinogen.

X   8-methoxypsoralen – see methoxsalen.

X   Methyl alcohol - mutagen; neurotoxin; skin and eye irritant; mild toxicity if inhaled; poison if swallowed; may cause blindness.

C   Methyl-alpha-d-glycopyranoside - skin irritant.

C   Methyl benzoate - has caused skin irritation in lab animals; toxic if ingested.

C   Methyl ester - see methyl benzoate.

C   Methyl gluceth - may contain toxic byproducts; see ethoxylated alcohols.

C   Methyl glucose sesquistearate - skin irritant; not adequately tested.

C   Methyl glucoside - skin and eye irritant; may be

harmful if inhaled or ingested; not adequately tested.

C A   3-methyl isothiazolin - can cause contact allergies.

CA   3-methyl isothiazolinone – see isothiazolinones.

CA   Methyl methacrylate – skin, eye and nail irritant; absorbed through skin, lungs, gastrointestinal tract; high level exposure may cause behavioral, neurochemical, bone marrow, brain kidney and liver changes; low level exposure can affect the liver; posssible heart and neurotoxic effects in occupationally exposed; developmental effects to fetus have occurred in lab animals; no reproductive studies have been performed; flammable.

†S   Methyl oleate - may cause acne; skin irritant.

C   Methyl salicylate – eye, skin and mucous membrane irritant; poison if swallowed; swallowing causes nausea, vomiting, shortness of breath; highly absorbable through skin; ingestion of small amounts has caused death; as of February 2000, CIR panel tentatively concluded this is safe when formulated to avoid irritation, and when formulated to avoid increasing sun sensitivity, if sun sensitivity is expected, directions should include use of sun protection.

†*S   Methylcellulose - skin and eye irritant.

†CA   Methylchloroisothiazolinone - preservative; strong allergen; CIR panel says safe with qualifications.

†CA   Methyldibromo glutaronitrile - preservative; skin irritant; skin absorbs readily; CIR panel says safe in "rinse-off" products, and up to .025% in "leave-on" products.

†CA   Methylisothiazolinone - preservative; strong allergen; CIR panel says safe with qualifications.

C A   2-methyl-4-isothiazolin-3-one - can cause allergies, contact dermatitis.

C   6-methylquinophthalone - can cause dermatitis.

CA   Methylparaben - preservative; mutagen; toxic if swallowed; may cause contact dermatitis; strong allergen.

CA   Methyl-p-hydroxybenzoate - see methylparaben.

CA   Methyl/propyl paraben – see methylparaben, propyl paraben.

X   7-methylpyrido[3,4-c]psoralen - phototoxic chemical, may damage DNA and cause mutations, tumors or neoplasms.

X   Methylene chloride – carcinogen; mutagen; may damage central nervous system, kidneys and liver; skin and eye irritant; inhalation causes headaches, tremors, nervousness, insomnia; banned in cosmetics.

φS   Mica – inhalation may damage lungs.

SA   Microcrystalline wax – petroleum derivative.

X   Mineral oil – petroleum derivative; phototoxin; eye and skin irritant; may cause acne, birth defects; potential carcinogen; may contain carcinogenic contaminants.

C   Mink oil – CIR Expert Panel says there is insufficient data to conclude it is safe.

CA   MIPA - see monoisopropanolamine.

C   Modulan - has caused tissue changes and skin irritation in lab animals.

C   Monoazoanilies - may cause acne.

†CA   Monoethanolamine – not studied for carcinogenic effects; CIR panel says safe up to 5% concentration in "rinse-off" products only; see ethanolamine.

CA   Monoethanolamine lauryl sulfate - may cause formation of carcinogens in products containing nitrogen compounds; contains ammonium salts; see ammonia, monoethanolamine.

CA   Monoethanolamine sulfite - skin irritant; contains ammonium salts; see ammonia, monoethanolamine.

CA   Monoisopropanolamine - skin and eye irritant; may cause formation of carcinogens in products containing nitrogen compounds.

CA   Monophenyl ether - can cause contact dermatitis, allergic reactions.

CA   Monotertiary butyl hydroquinone - can cause contact dermatitis, allergic reactions.

X   Mountain savory – essential oil; severe skin and mucous membrane irritant; never use undiluted; exercise extreme caution; avoid if pregnant.

*XA   MSG - may cause headaches, itching, nausea, brain, nervous system, reproductive disorders, high blood pressure; pregnant, lactating mothers, infants, small children should avoid; allergic reactions common; may be hidden in cosmetics, hair conditioners, shampoos, soaps, infant formula, low fat milk, candy, chewing gum, drinks, over-the-counter medications, especially children's, binders and fillers for nutritional supplements, prescription and non-prescription drugs, IV fluids given in hospitals, chicken pox vaccine; it is being sprayed on growing fruits and vegetables as a growth enhancer; it is proposed for use on organic crops.

SA   Musk - may cause allergic reactions.

*CA   Musk ambrette - causes photosensitivity; skin irritant; may damage myelin nerve coverings.

SA   Musk moskene - may cause skin hyperpigmention; skin irritant.

C   Mustard oil - essential oil; burns the skin if used improperly; avoid if allergies or nervous conditions.

CA   Myristamidopropyl dimethylamine - skin irritant; potentially toxic.

C   Myristates - may cause acne; may be toxic.

†CA   Myristic acid - skin irritant; mutagen.

C   Myristica fragrans – see nutmeg oil.

†SA   Myristyl alcohol - skin irritant.

†S   Myristyl myristate - may cause acne.

S   Myristyl propionate - may cause acne.

*Cl   Myrrh – see myrrh oil.

*Cl   Myrrh oil - essential oil; antiseptic; antifungal; immune stimulant; circulatory stimulant; uterine stimulant; avoid if pregnant or lactating; see essential oils.

S   Myrtle – essential oil; astringent; anti-bacterial; anti-inflammatory; see essential oils.

S   Myrtus communis – see myrtle.

†C   NaPCA – may cause the formation of carcinogenic
         nitrosamines if product contains nitrogen compounds;
         otherwise CIR considers safe.

CA   Naphtha – petroleum derivative; skin irritant; may
         cause dry skin, difficulty breathing, dizziness.

XA   Naphthalene - coal tar derivative; skin and eye
         irritant; poison; potential carcinogen; neurotoxin.

XA   Naphthol – coal tar derivative; skin and eye irritant;
         poison; see coal tar derivatives.

S   Nardostachys jatamansi – see spikenard.

S   Natural essence oils – see natural oils.

S   Natural oils – if cold pressed, contain substances
         beneficial for the skin; if solvent extracted or hot
         pressed, they are highly refined and most beneficial
         substances are destroyed.

CA   Natural fragrance – potential sensitizer; may cause
         allergic dermatitis.

C   n-butyl benzoate - skin irritant in rabbits.

XA   Neomycin - antibacterial; toxic to kidneys; may
         affect hearing; has caused resistant strains of
         staphylococcus bacteria to develop; skin irritant.

S   Neroli oil - essential oil; antiseptic; anti-bacterial;
         anti-viral; see essential oils.

S   Nettle – herb; healing properties; anti-aging.

S   Niacin - see vitamin B3.

XA   Nickel - skin irritant; may cause asthma, depression,
         kidney and brain damage; carcinogen; mutagen.

XA   Nickel sulfate - skin irritant; may cause depression,
         kidney and brain damage; potential carcinogen;
         contains ammonium salts, see ammonia.

C   Niobe oil - see methyl benzoate.

X   Nitrilotriacetic acid - irritant; possible carcinogen.

X   o-nitro-p-aminophenol – carcinogen.

X   Nitrobenzene - toxic if inhaled, ingested or absorbed
         through the skin; poison; possible carcinogen.

X   4-nitro-o-phenylenediamine - mutagen, may cause
         genetic damage; not adequately tested.

X   <u>2-nitrophenylenediamine</u> - mutagen, may cause genetic damage.

X   <u>2-nitro-4-phenylenediamine</u> - carcinogen, mutagen, may cause genetic damage.

X   <u>2-nitropropane</u> – possible carcinogen.

X   <u>Nitrosamines</u> – carcinogens; contains ammonium salts, see ammonia.

X   <u>n-nitroso compounds</u> - carcinogenic cosmetic contaminant; contains ammonium salts, see ammonia.

X   <u>n-nitroso-n-methylalkylamines</u> - carcinogenic contaminant; contains ammonium salts, see ammonia.

X   <u>n-nitroso-n-methyltetradecyl amine</u> - carcinogenic contaminant; contains ammonium salts, see ammonia.

X   <u>n-nitrosoalkanolamines</u> – carcinogen; contains ammonium salts, see ammonia.

X   <u>n-nitrosobis(2-hydroxypropyl)amine</u> – carcinogen; contains ammonium salts, see ammonia.

X   <u>n-nitrosodiethanolamine</u> - carcinogenic cosmetic contaminant; easily absorbed through skin; contains ammonium salts, see ammonia.

X   <u>n-nitrosodimethylamine</u> - carcinogenic cosmetic contaminant; contains ammonium salts, see ammonia.

X   <u>n-nitrosomorpholine</u> - carcinogenic cosmetic contaminant; contains ammonium salts, see ammonia.

X   <u>Nonylphenol</u> –toxic if skin contact and if swallowed; toxic to endocrine system; not adequately tested.

X   <u>4-NOPD</u> - mutagen, may cause genetic damage.

CA   <u>Novocain</u> - skin irritant; may cause swelling, anxiety, asthma; respiratory arrest.

C   <u>n-propyl benzoate</u> – causes inflammation in rabbits.

C   <u>n-propylamines</u> - strong skin irritant; hazardous.

C   <u>Nutmeg oil</u> - essential oil; antiseptic; anti-inflammatory; undiluted may cause convulsions and increased heart rate; avoid if pregnant; see essential oils.

C   Nutrient additives - nutrients added to mostly refined and processed foods giving a false sense of nutritional value and can lead to nutritional imbalances; chemicals used in preparing nutrients added are not listed on the label.

SA   Oak moss - skin irritant.

SA   1-octadecanol – see stearyl alcohol.

SA   Octadecyl alcohol – see stearyl alcohol.

CA   Octhilinone – see Kathon CG.

X   Octocrylene – see phenol.

C   Octyl dimethyl PABA - may cause formation of nitrosamines; not adequately tested.

XA   Octyl methoxycinnamate – skin irritant; not tested for safety.

†S   Octyl palmitate - may cause acne.

C   Octyl salicylate – see salicylic acid.

†S   Octyl stearate - may cause acne.

XA   Octylacrylamide/acrylates/butylaminoethyl methacrylate copolymer – causes allergic reactions if inhaled; may contain hydroquinone benzoyl peroxide; see hydroquinone and benzoyle peroxide.

XA   Octylacrylamide/acrylates/butylaminoethyl methacrylate polymer - causes allergic reactions if inhaled; may contain hydroquinone benzoyl peroxide; see hydroquinone and benzoyle peroxide.

C   Octyoxynol-n - may contain toxic byproducts.

S   Oils – must be cold pressed to preserve any healing and beneficial properties; heat pressed or solvent-extracted oils are highly refined and have lost healing and beneficial properties; see specific oil.

†SA   Oil of jojoba – see jojoba oil, oils.

S   Oil of kuawa – oil of guava; many healing properties; see oils.

S   Oil of kukui – candlenut oil; carrier oil mixed with essential oils; see oils.

*CA   Oil of lemongrass - essential oil; skin irritant; insect repellant; anti-fungal; antibacterial; mildly toxic if swallow large amounts; see lemongrass oil, essential oils.

S   Oil of lilikoi –passion fruit oil; see oils.

S   Oil of manako –mango oil; see oils.

SA   Oil of mikana –papaya oil; see oils.

X   Oil of mirbane - see nitrobenzene; see oils.

*C1   Oil of myrrh - essential oil; see myrrh oil, essential oils.

CA   Oil of orange – see orange oil; essential oils.

S   Oil of orchid - see oils.

S   Oil of plumeria – essential oil from tropical flower.

C   Oil of purcellin - skin irritant.

S   Oil of Taro – oil of Polynesian root vegetable.

†S   Oil of wheat germ

C   Oil of wintergreen – see methyl salicylate.

†CA   Oleamide DEA – may cause formation of carcinogens in products containing nitrogen compounds; mucous membrane and skin irritant; CIR panel says safe up to 10% concentrations in products that do not contain nitrosating agents; see DEA.

CA   Oleamidopropyl dimethylamine - skin irritant; may be toxic.

†CA   Oleic acid - skin irritant; may cause acne; mutagen; potential carcinogen.

†C   Oleth-n - may contain dangerous byproducts; see ethoxylated alcohols.

S   Oleyl alcohol

SA   Olive oil - may cause acne.

X   o-benzene dicarboxylic acid; see phthalic acid.

X   o-nitro-p-aminophenol – carcinogen.

X   o-phenylenediamine - carcinogen; mutagen.

X   o-phthalic acid –see phthalic acid.

*CA   Orange bitter – see orange oil.

S   Orange blossom oil – see neroli oil.

*CA   Orange essence – see orange oil.

*CA   Orange oil – essential oil; astringent; antibacterial; skin irritant; may cause photosensitivity; frequent use or inhalation may cause shortness of breath, dizziness, headaches; possible carcinogen; see essential oils.

C   <u>Oregano oil</u> – essential oil; antiseptic; anti-bacterial; anti-fungal; severe skin irritant; see essential oils.

*C   <u>Origanum oil</u> - essential oil; skin irritant; avoid if pregnant or lactating; ingestion may cause illness or death; use in minute amounts; see essential oils.

C   <u>Origanum compactum</u> – see oregano oil.

C1   <u>Origanum majorana</u> – see marjoram oil.

CA   <u>Orris oil</u> - essential oil; frequent allergen; purgative; causes asthma, hay fever, stuffy nose, red eyes, infantile eczema, nausea and vomiting; toxic.

C   <u>Other ingredients</u> – ingredients not required to be listed on the label; may or may not be harmful; may be contaminated with carcinogens or other harmful chemicals.

X   <u>Oxirane</u> - see ethylene oxide.

CA   <u>Oxybenzone</u> - may cause photosensitivity; skin irritant.

XA   <u>Oxymethylene</u> - see formaldehyde.

CA   <u>PABA</u> – component of vitamin B; sunscreen; prevents sunburn and may prevent skin cancer; may cause contact dermatitis and photo sensitivity in sensitive individuals.

X   <u>p-acetylphenetidin</u> – see phenacetin.

C   <u>Padimate-O</u> – may cause formation of nitrosamines; not adequately tested.

S   <u>Palmarosa oil</u> - essential oil; antiseptic, anti-bacterial; antifungal; antiviral; see essential oils.

†C   <u>Palmitate</u> - possible skin irritant; adverse reactions.

†SA   <u>Palmitic acid</u> - may irritate skin.

SA   <u>Palmityl alcohol</u> - may cause skin irritation.

CA   <u>P-aminobenzoic acid</u> - see PABA.

CA   <u>Para aminobenzoic acid</u> – see PABA.

C1   <u>Panax ginseng</u> – herb; demulcent; stimulant; may increase cell life; may cause vaginal bleeding; avoid if asthma, cardiac arrhythmia, clotting problems, emphysema, fever, high blood pressure, pregnant; do not give to children.

S   Pantothenic acid - vitamin B5; beneficial for hair; see nutrient additives.

S   Panthenol - B vitamin.

CA   Parabens - may irritate skin; may be toxic if swallowed; potential mutagen.

C   Paraffin – may contain carcinogens.

†X   Paraphenylenediamine – see phenylenediamine.

X   Paraphenylenediamine dihydrochloride– see phenylenediamine.

CA   Parsley oil - essential oil; skin irritant; toxic in strong doses; stimulates the nervous system; phototoxic; may cause miscarriage.

CA   Parsley seed oil – see parsley oil

SA   Patchouli oil - essential oil; antiseptic; anti-fungal; may irritate the chemically sensitive; see essential oils.

SA   Peanut oil – may cause acne.

C   PEG – eye and skin irritant; hazardous on large areas of the body; may be contaminated with dangerous levels of 1,4-dioxane, a carcinogen; see ethoxylated alcohols.

C   PEG-n (4-200) – see PEG.

†C   PEG-6 – CIR panel says safe, but should not be used on damaged skin; see PEG.

†C   PEG-20 – see PEG-6.

†C   PEG-75 – see PEG-6.

C   PEG-2M - may be contaminated with dangerous levels of 1,4-dioxane, a carcinogen; see ethoxylated alcohols.

C   PEG 90M - may be contaminated with dangerous levels of 1,4-dioxane, a carcinogen; see ethoxylated alcohols.

C   PEG-n cocamine – CIR panel says insufficient data to support safety.

CA   PEG-n lanolin – see PEG, lanolin.

C   PEG –n soy sterol - CIR panel says insufficient data

to support safety.

C   PEG-n stearate – see PEG.

C   PEG/PPG 17/6 copolymer - may be contaminated with dangerous levels of 1,4-dioxane, a carcinogen; see ethoxylated alcohols.

SA   Pelargonium graveolens – see geranium oil.

†C1A   Peppermint oil - essential oil; antiseptic; anti-inflammatory; may cause hay fever, skin irritation; frequent use may cause contact sensitization; use with caution or avoid if pregnant or high blood pressure; see essential oils.

X   Perchloroethylene – see tetrachloroethylene.

CA   Perfumes - may cause skin irritation, headaches, dizziness, coughing, vomiting, hyperpigmentation.

S   Persulphates – may irritate skin and mucous membranes; contains ammonium salts, see ammonia.

CA   Peruvian balsam – see balsam of Peru.

X   Perylene – carcinogen.

X   p-ethoxyacetanilide – see phenacetin.

S   Petitgrain – essential oil; antiseptic; anti-bacterial; anti-inflammatory; see essential oils.

CA   Petrolatum – petroleum derivative; may contain carcinogenic contaminants; may cause acne.

CA   Petroleum distillates – see naphtha.

X   Phenacetin – severe skin irritant; carcinogen; mutagen; toxic if ingested.

X   Phenol – coal tar derivative; toxic if inhaled, swallowed or absorbed through the skin; ingestion of 1.5 grams or .05 ounce has caused death; absorption through skin can cause death.

†XA   Phenoxyethanol - eye irritant undiluted; non-irritating at 2.2% dilution or less; can cause contact dermatitis; suspected teratogen; not adequately tested.

†XA   2-phenoxyethanol – see phenoxyethanol.

†S   Phenyl trimethicone – CIR panel says safe as used in cosmetics.

XA   Phenylenediamine – skin irritant; has caused cancer in some lab animals; mutagen; may cause asthma, genetic damage; photosensitizer; can be absorbed through the skin; currently on CIR top priority list to study for safety.

XA   1,2-phenylenediamine – see phenylenediamine.

†XA   m-phenylenediamine - see phenylenediamine.

XA   o-phenylenediamine - see phenylenediamine.

XA   p-phenylenediamine - see phenylenediamine.

CA   Phenylformic acid - skin irritant, harmful if ingested.

XA   Phenylmercuric acetate – skin irritant; extremely toxic; contains mercury.

C   Phenylmethanol - may cause contact dermatitis.

C   3-Phenylpropenal - see cinnamic aldehyde.

*C   Phosphoric acid – skin, eye, nose, throat and respiratory irritant; corrosive; skin contact and swallowing are moderately toxic.

X   Phthalates – carcinogenic; mutagenic; may adversely affect sperm.

X   Phthalic acid – mucous membrane and skin irritant; see phthalates.

S   Picea alba – see spruce oil.

S   Picea mariana – see spruce oil.

CA   Pigments – insoluble uncertified color additives; most are azo dyes or coal tar dyes which are carcinogenic; e.g. Pigment Red 4.

CA   Pinene – skin irritant; constituent of pine oil; see pine oil.

CA   Pine oil - essential oil; antiseptic; anti-bacterial; anti-viral; skin and mucous membrane irritant; central nervous system depressant in large doses; see essential oils.

CA   Pinus sylvestris – see pine oil.

S   Plantago – herb; astringent, heals allergies and skin.

S   Plantain – herb; astringent, heals allergies and skin.

SA   Pogostemon cablin – see patchouli oil.

SA   Pogostemon patchouli – see patchouli oil.

X   Polycylic aromatic hydrocarbons (PAH) – carcinogen.

C   Polyether glycol – see PEG.

C	<u>Polyethoxylated compounds</u> – may contain carcinogen 1,4-dioxane; see ethoxylated alcohols.
C	<u>Polyethylene glycol</u> – can break down into formaldehyde; see PEG, formaldehyde.
C	<u>Polyglycol</u> – see PEG.
CA	<u>Polymethyl methacrylate</u> – eye, skin and respiratory irritant; possible carcinogen.
CA	<u>Polyols</u> – see polyethylene glycol, propylene glycol.
C	<u>Polyoxethylene compounds</u> – may be contaminated with carcinogenic 1,4-dioxane; see ethoxylated alcohols.
C	<u>Polyoxyethylene sorbitan monooleate</u> – skin irritant; may be contaminated with carcinogenic 1,4-dioxane; see ethoxylated alcohols.
†CA	<u>Polypropylene glycol</u> – skin and eye irritant; slightly toxic on skin contact; hazardous on large areas of the body; CIR panel says safe up to 50% concentration.
XA	<u>Polyquaternium-10</u> – see quaternary ammonium compounds.
†S	<u>Polysorbate (1-85)</u> – skin irritant.
†C	<u>Polysorbate-60</u> – may be contaminated with carcinogen 1,4-dioxane; see ethoxylated alcohols.
†C	<u>Polysorbate-80</u> – may be contaminated with carcinogen 1,4-dioxane; see ethoxylated alcohols.
†XA	<u>Polyvinyl acetate</u> – see polyvinylpyrrolidone.
†XA	<u>Polyvinylpyrrolidone</u> – petroleum derivative; may cause gas, constipation, lung and kidney damage; may cause foreign bodies in lungs from breathing in hairspray containing this ingredient.
†S	<u>Potassium cocohydrolyzed protein</u>
C	<u>Potassium hydroxide</u> – severe skin and eye irritant; has caused tumors on skin of mice; ingestion can be fatal.
φS	<u>Potassium sodium copper chlorophyllin</u> – only for use in toothpaste or tooth powder; must be used according to specific requirements.
†C	<u>Potassium sorbate</u> – skin irritant, may be mutagenic; mildly toxic if swallowed.

†C   <u>PPG</u> – see polypropylene glycol.

C   <u>PPG-2-isodeceth-4</u> – may contain carcinogenic contaminants; see ethoxylated alcohols.

C   <u>PPG-m ceteth-n</u> – may be contaminated with carcinogens; see ethoxylated alcohols.

CA   <u>Procaine</u> - see novocain.

CA   <u>Procaine hydrochloride</u> - see novocain.

†C   <u>Propane</u> – propellant; neurotoxin at high concentrations; flammable.

†CA   <u>1,2-propanediol</u> – see polypropylene glycol.

CA   <u>Propanediols</u> – skin irritant; causes unilateral pupil dilation; may cause delayed allergic reaction.

*S   <u>1,2,3-propanetriol</u> - see glycerol.

C   <u>Propantheline bromide</u> – causes unilateral pupil dilation.

†S   <u>Propolis</u> – skin irritant.

†CA   <u>Propyl gallate</u> – skin irritant; suspected carcinogen; associated with kidney, liver problems, gastrointestinal irritation; has caused cancer in laboratory animals; not adequately tested; CIR panel says safe as used in cosmetics.

CA   <u>Propyl paraben</u> - skin irritant; low toxicity; may cause contact dermatitis; strong allergen.

CA   <u>Propyl-p-hydroxybenzoate</u> – see propylparaben.

CA   <u>Propylamine</u> – causes skin irritation, contact dermatitis.

†CA   <u>Propylene glycol</u> - petrochemical, best avoided; absorbs quickly through skin; strong irritant; may cause delayed allergic reaction, acne, contact dermatitis; see polypropylene glycol.

C   <u>Propylene glycol ceteth-n</u> – may contain carcinogenic contaminants; see ethoxylated alcohols.

S   <u>Propylene glycol-2 myristyl propionate</u> – may cause acne.

CA   <u>Propylparaben</u> – preservative; skin irritant; low toxicity; strong allergen; may cause contact dermatitis.

X   <u>Psoralen</u> - phototoxic chemical; may damage DNA

and cause mutations, tumors or neoplasms.

S Purified water

†XA PVP – see polyvinylpyrrolidone.

S Pyridoxine - see vitamin B6.

X Pyrocatechol - CIR panel determined this ingredient to be unsafe for leave-on products; insufficient data available to assure safety for use in hair dyes.

φC Pyrophyllite – aluminum compound of anhydrous aluminum silicate and silica; aluminum has been linked to Alzheimer's; see external use only.

XA Quaternary ammonium compounds - extremely toxic; skin and eye irritant; cause hair to become dry and brittle with long-term use; may cause anaphalytic shock.

†XA Quaternarium - 15 - causes dermatitis; skin and eye irritant; may cause birth defects; releases formaldehyde; teratogenic effects in rats; sensitizer; see formaldehyde.

CA Quaternarium-18 – skin and eye irritant; sensitizer.

C Quinaldine – strong mucous membrane irritant; harmful if absorbed through skin; moderate health hazard.

XA Quinol - see hydroquinone.

XA Quinoline yellow – skin irritant; causes dermatitis; derived from coal tar, a carcinogen.

XA Quinolines – skin irritant; causes dermatitis; derived from coal tar, a carcinogen.

XA Quinophthalone – see solvent yellow 33.

S Ravensara – essential oil; antiseptic; anti-bacterial; anti-viral; anti-fungal; see essential oils.

S Ravensara aromatica – see ravensara.

XA Red No. 3 – carcinogen; banned for cosmetics and drugs used externally; still approved for use in foods and drugs taken internally

φXA Red No. 4 – causes atrophied adrenal glands and bladder polyps in animals, banned in food and drugs, but allowed in cosmetics; see external use only

C Red No. 36 – skin irritant; causes acne.

φXA Red No. 40 – see FD&C Red No. 40.

φXA Red No. 40 Lake – see FD&C Red No. 40 aluminum lake.

†CA Red oil - see oleic acid.

SA Red petrolatum – may cause skin discoloration; derived from petroleum.

†CA Resorcinol – causes contact dermatitis; when using, avoid acne preparations, alcohol- containing products, medicated cosmetics, abrasive cleansers and soaps; FDA states resorcinol not shown safe and effective as claimed in over-the-counter products.

X Resorcinolphthalein - see fluoresceins.

*S Retinol - beneficial for skin; see vitamin A.

†S Retinyl palmitate - see vitamin A.

C Rhodamine B – interferes with collagen synthesis on the lips; inhibits cellular metabolism of the skin.

C Rhodamines – inhibits cellular metabolism of the skin.

S Riboflavin - see vitamin B2.

*CA Ricinoleamidopropyl dimethylamine lactate – corrosive to skin, eyes, throat, nose; toxic by skin contact and if swallowed.

C Ricinoleic acid – skin irritant; potential carcinogen.

CA Ricinus oil - see castor oil.

S Rosa damascena – see rose oil.

S Rosa rubiginosa – see rosehip oil.

S Rosalina – essential oil; anti-bacterial; anti-fungal; heating causes loss of therapeutic value; see essential oils.

S Rose oil - essential oil; anti-infectious; aphrodisiac; use cautiously or avoid if pregnant; see essential oils.

S Rose centifolia – see rose oil.

S Rose damascena – see rose oil.

S Rose geranium oil - essential oil

S Rosehip oil – essential oil; healing for skin conditions; see essential oils.

*C1 Rosemarinus officinalis – see rosemary oil..

*C1A Rosemary extract – may cause skin irritation,

74

photosensitivity; avoid if pregnant, epileptic, high blood pressure; see extract.

*C1   Rosemary oil - essential oil; antiseptic; astringent; avoid if pregnant, epileptic, high blood pressure; see essential oils.

S   Rosewood oil - essential oil; anti-bacterial; anti-viral; anti-fungal; see essential oils.

CA   Rosin - skin irritant.

*C1   Rosmarinus officinalis – see rosemary oil.

CA   Rue oil – may cause photosensitivity; on FDA list to investigate for reproductive, mutagenic and teratogenic effects.

X   Saccharin – potential carcinogen; currently being evaluated by National Toxicology Program.

†S   Safflower oil – deep moisturizer; may irritate skin; may cause acne; see oils.

C1   Sage – herb; astringent; antiseptic; disinfectant; avoid if pregnant, epileptic, high blood pressure.

C1   Sage oil - essential oil; astringent; antiseptic; disinfectant; avoid if pregnant, epileptic, high blood pressure; toxic if taken internally; see essential oils.

C1A   St. Johnswort – see hypericum perforatum.

C   Salicylic acid – eye and skin irritant; poison if swallowed; large amounts absorbed through skin may cause abdominal pain, vomiting, tinnitis, mental disturbances; mutagen.

C1   Salvia officinalis – see sage oil.

C1   Salvia sclarea – see clary sage.

S   Sandalwood oil - essential oil; antiseptic; astringent; see essential oils.

S   Santalum album – see sandalwood oil.

C   Sassafras oil - essential oil; toxic; suspected carcinogen.

X   Satureja montana – see mountain savory.

CA   Scoparone – see coumarin.

SA   Scotch pine – herb; essential oil; fragrance; skin irritant.

C   SD alcohol – see denatured alcohol.

C   SD alcohol 40 – see denatured alcohol.

C   SD alcohol 40 – 8 – see denatured alcohol.

S   Seed of plantago - herb, antibacterial, anti-fungal.

C   Selenium sulfide – severe eye and skin irritant.

S   Sesame oil – may cause acne; see oils.

CA   Sesquiterpine lactone – naturally occurring component of essential oils; may cause severe allergies.

C   Silica – toxic if inhaled or swallowed; may be contaminated with crystalline quartz, a carcinogen; see external use only.

CA   Silk powder – may cause hives; systemic symptoms if ingested or inhaled.

φC   Silver – mucous membrane and skin irritant; skin discoloration may result from prolonged absorption; limited to fingernail polish.

XA   Soapstone – see talc

†CA   Sodium benzoate – skin irritant; toxic if swallowed; avoid if asthma or liver problems; may cause hyperactivity in children; CIR panel says safe in concentrations up to 5%, insufficient data to support safety in products where exposure involves inhalation.

*XA   Sodium bisulfite – strong skin, eye and mucous membrane irritant; corrosive; mutagen; may cause asthma, anaphylactic shock; contains ammonium salts, see ammonia.

*S   Sodium chloride – eye and skin irritant.

†C   Sodium cocoyl sarcosinate – CIR panel says safe in "rinse-off" products as used, safe in "leave-on" products up to 5% concentration, insufficient data to determine safety in products where ingredient may be inhaled, may cause formation of carcinogenic nitrosamines in products containing nitrogen compounds.

*C   Sodium dioctyl sulfosuccinate – skin and eye irritant; moderately toxic.

CA   Sodium dodecyl sulfate – skin irritant; may cause

eczema; contains ammonium salts, see ammonia.

†CA   Sodium dodecylbenzene sulfonate – skin and eye irritant; has caused liver, kidney and intestinal damage when ingested by animals.

X   Sodium fluoride – see fluoride.

X   Sodium hydroxide – severe eye and skin irritant; corrosive; mutagen.

†C   Sodium laureth sulfate - skin and eye irritant; may be contaminated with dangerous levels of toxins; contains ammonium salts; see ammonia, ethoxylated alcohols.

†C   Sodium laureth-n sulfate - see sodium laureth sulfate.

†C   Sodium lauroyl sarcosinate – see sodium cocoyl sarcosinate.

†CA   Sodium lauryl sulfate – may cause dry skin, eczema; skin irritant; mutagen; CIR panel says safe as used in "rinse-off" products, up to 1% concentration in "leave-on" products; contains ammonium salts, see ammonia.

C   Sodium oleth sulfate - may be contaminated with dangerous levels of toxins; contains ammonium salts; see ammonia, ethoxylated alcohols.

†C   Sodium PCA – see NaPCA.

S   Sodium phosphate – skin and eye irritant.

X   Sodium saccharin – see saccharin.

C   Sodium silicate – skin, eye and mucous membrane irritant; corrosive; poison if swallowed.

†CA   Sodium stearate – 93% stearic acid; see stearic acid.

†C   Sodium sulfate – skin eye and respiratory irritant; corrosive; may trigger asthma attacks; CIR says safe for rinse-off products and a maximum concentration of 1% in leave-on products; contains ammonium salts, see ammonia.

C   Sodium trideceth sulfate - may be contaminated with dangerous levels of toxins; see ethoxylated alcohols; contains ammonium salts, see ammonia.

*X   Sodiumsulphosuccinate – eye, mucous membrane

and skin irritant; potentially harmful if absorbed through skin, inhaled or swallowed; not adequately tested.

CA   <u>Solvent dyes</u> – uncertified colors; most are azo dyes or coal tar dyes which are carcinogenic; e.g. Solvent Green 3.

XA   <u>Solvent yellow 33</u> – coal tar dye; see D&C Yellow No. 11, quinolines.

†C   <u>Sorbic acid</u> –causes hives; skin irritant; mutagen; mildly toxic if swallowed.

C   <u>Sorbitan laurate</u> –causes hives.

C   <u>Sorbitan oleate</u> –causes hives.

C   <u>Sorbitan palmitate</u> –causes hives.

C   <u>Sorbitan sequioleate</u> –causes hives.

C   <u>Sorbitan stearate</u> – may cause hives.

*SA   <u>Sorbitol</u> – no known toxicity for external use; taken internally, may cause gastrointestinal distress, may change rate of absorption of drugs.

SA   <u>Soy protein</u> – may be genetically modified; may cause allergic acne.

C1   <u>Spearmint oil</u> - essential oil; antiseptic; anti-bacterial; anti-fungal; avoid on infants and small children; use cautiously or avoid if pregnant; see essential oils.

S   <u>Spikenard</u> – skin tonic; anti-bacterial, anti-fungal; see essential oils.

S   <u>Spruce oil</u> - essential oil; anti-inflammatory; disinfectant; see essential oils.

CA   <u>Starch</u> – may cause stuffy nose if inhaled; blocks pores on skin.

CA   <u>Stearamidoethyl diethylamine phosphate</u> – skin and mucous membrane irritant.

CA   <u>Stearamidopropyl dimethylamine</u> – skin and mucous membrane irritant; may be carcinogenic.

C   <u>Stearamin oxyd</u> – may cause formation of carcinogenic nitrosamines.

†C   <u>Stearamine oxide</u> - may cause formation of carcinogenic nitrosamines; CIR panel says safe for "rinse-off" products and up to 5% concentration in

"leave-on" products.

†C   Steareth-n - may be contaminated with dangerous levels of toxins; see ethoxylated alcohols.

†SA   Stearic acid – skin irritant; potential sensitizer; may cause acne.

SA   Stearyl alcohol – skin irritant.

XA   Steatite – see talc.

S   Stinging nettle – see nettle.

SA   Styrax benzoin - essential oil; see benzoin.

S   Sucrose cocoate

CA   Sulfanilamide – antibacterial; toxic.

CA   Sulfur – skin, eye and respiratory irritant; banned in products for cold sores, fever blisters and diaper rash; FDA says not shown safe in products for treating lice, poison oak, poison ivy and poison sumac.

†C   Sulisobenzone – see benzophenone.

S   Sunflower oil – see oils.

CA   Sweet birch oil – see birch oil.

C   Sweet fennel oil - essential oil; anti-inflammatory; antiseptic; diuretic; skin sensitizer; possible carcinogen; epileptics should not use; avoid during pregnancy.

S   Sweet orange oil - essential oil; may cause dermatitis.

C   Symphytum officinalis – see comfrey.

φS   Synthetic iron oxides

XA   Talc – possible skin and lung irritant; toxic if inhaled; carcinogen; never use on babies.

XA   Talcum – see talc.

XA   Talcum powder – may cause vomiting, coughing, pneumonia in babies if inhaled; increases risk of ovarian cancer if used on sanitary napkins or genitals; see talc.

C   Tanacetum vulgare – see wild tansy oil.

S   Tangerine oil – anti-inflammatory; may cause photosensitivity; see essential oils.

C1   Tarragon oil – essential oil; antiseptic; anti-bacterial; anti-viral; avoid if pregnant, epileptic; see essential oils.

†C   TEA – skin, mucous membrane and eye irritant; causes contact dermatitis; sensitizer; may cause formation of carcinogenic nitrosamines in products containing nitrogen compounds; may contain nitrosamine contaminants not listed on the label; mildly toxic if swallowed; CIR panel says safe up to 5% concentration in "rinse-off" products only.

C   TEA carbomer – see TEA.

C   TEA coco hydrolyzed protein – severe skin irritant; see TEA.

C   TEA cocoyl glutamate – see TEA, glutamic acid.

†C   TEA lauryl sulfate – contains ammonium salts; see ammonia, TEA, sodium lauryl sulfate.

C   TEA salicylate - phototoxic chemical; in sunlight may cause formation of carcinogenic nitrosamines; see salicylic acid, TEA.

†CA   TEA stearate – see TEA, stearic acid.

S   Tea tree oil - see melaleuca alternifolia.

†CA   Tektamer 38 - see methyldibromo glutaronitrile.

SA   Terpenes – may cause facial psoriasis.

C A   2-tert-butylhydroquinone - can cause contact dermatitis.

XA   Tertiary ammonium compounds – skin irritant; may cause anaphylactic shock

X   Tetrachloroethylene – skin, eye and respiratory irritant; dries skin; neurotoxin; probable carcinogen.

SA   1-tetradecanol - see myristyl alcohol

CA   Tetrahydronaphthalene – skin, eye and respiratory irritant; may cause severe dermatitis, liver and kidney damage; central nervous system depressant; neurotoxin.

X   2,4,5,7-tetraiodofluorescein disodium salt – coal tar color; carcinogen.

CA   Tetrasodium EDTA – see disodium EDTA.

CA   Tetrasodium salt – see disodium EDTA.

SA   Theobroma oil - see cocoa butter.

†CA   Thioglycolic acid – severe allergen, skin irritant; causes hair to break; see ammonium thioglycolate.

X   Thiomersal – preservative in eye cosmetics and vaccines given to infants; skin irritant; contains mercury, which has been banned in cosmetics except in eye cosmetics because of mercury buildup; small amounts ingested can be fatal.

CA   Thyme extract – skin and mucous membrane irritant; may cause hay fever; avoid if pregnant, high blood pressure, thyroid problems.

C   Thyme oil - essential oil; antiseptic; antibacterial, anti-viral; anti-fungal; skin and mucous membrane irritant; avoid if pregnant, high blood pressure, thyroid problems; see essential oils.

C   Thymus vulgaris – see thyme oil.

φS   Titanium dioxide – may irritate skin; inhalation of large amounts of titanium dioxide dust may cause lung damage.

SA   Tocopherol (vitamin E) – antioxidant; healing to skin; may cause contact dermatitis; may be soy, peanut, corn based; may be natural or synthetic; see nutrient additives.

SA   Tocopherol acetate (vitamin E) – see tocopherol.

SA   Tocopheryl acetate (vitamin E) – longer shelf life, but cannot be utilized by the skin.

†C   Toluene – coal tar derivative; skin, eye and respiratory irritant; neurotoxin; may cause asthma and trigger attacks; high concentrations may cause death; repeated inhalation may cause permanent brain damage; adverse effects worsened if consume alcohol at time of exposure, or suffer from kidney, liver or skin disorders; classified as hazardous by OSHA; CIR panel says safe as used in cosmetics.

X   Toluene-2,4-diamine - see 2,4-diaminotoluene.

X   2,4-toluenediamine – see 2,4-diaminotoluene.

X   m-toluenediamine - mutagen, carcinogen.

†CA   Toluenesulfonamide formaldehyde resin – skin irritant; strong sensitizer when liquid; causes contact dermatitis.

CA   Tonka bean - see coumarin.

CA   Tonka bean camphor - see coumarin.

XA   Tricetylmonium chloride – see quaternary ammonium compounds.

X   Trichloroethane – eye, skin and mucous membrane irritant; neurotoxin; not adequately tested for carcinogenicity; narcotic in high amounts; may adversely affect the heart, including cardiac arrest.

X   1,1,1-tricholorethane – see tricholorethane.

CA   Triclosan – skin irritant; may cause contact dermatitis, liver damage; mutagen; moderately toxic on skin contact and if swallowed.

†C   Triethanolamine - see TEA.

C   Triethanolamine salts – eye and skin irritant; see TEA.

†X   Triisopropanolamine – severe eye, skin, mucous membrane, upper respiratory tract irritant; harmful if absorbed through skin, inhaled or swallowed; not adequately tested; CIR panel says safe with qualifications.

X   4,5,8-trimethylpsoralen - phototoxic chemical, may damage DNA and cause mutations, tumors or neoplasms.

S   Tropaeolum majus – herb; antibacterial; antifungal.

XA   Turpentine oil – nose, throat and skin irritant; may cause headaches, hallucinations, kidney and lung damage, death; depresses central nervous system.

φS   Ultramarine blue – see "external use only."

φS   Ultramarine green – see "external use only."

φS   Ultramarine pink – see "external use only."

φS   Ultramarine red – see "external use only."

φS   Ultramarine violet – see "external use only."

*CA   Urea – skin irritant; mutagen.

X   Urocanic acid – phototoxin; not adequately tested; avoid if using alpha-hydroxy acids; CIR panel says insufficient data to support safety.

S   Urtica dioica – see nettle.

C   Vaccinium myrtillus – see bilberry.

C   <u>Valerates</u> – skin irritant; suspected carcinogen.

S   <u>Valerian oil</u> – essential oil; anti-bacterial; central
         nervous system depressant; frequent use may cause
         contact sensitization; see essential oils.

S   <u>Valeriana officinalis</u> – see valerian oil.

C   <u>Valeric acid</u> – eye, throat, nose and skin irritant;
         moderately toxic if inhaled or swallowed.

C   <u>Vanillin</u> – skin irritant; sensitizer; causes burning
         sensation, contact dermatitis, eczema, skin
         pigmentation.

SA   <u>Vegetable emulsifying wax</u>

S   <u>Verbena oil</u> – causes photosensitivity; see oils.

C1   <u>Vetiver oil</u> - essential oil; antiseptic; use cautiously or
         avoid if pregnant; see essential oils.

C1   <u>Vetiveria zizanoides</u> – see veviter oil.

C   <u>Vinyl acetate/crotonic acid/vinyl neodecanoate
         polymer</u> - toxic if inhaled

SA   <u>Violet oil</u> - essential oil; antiseptic; anti-
         inflammatory; high doses can cause diarrhea and
         vomiting.

*S   <u>Vitamin A</u> - important for the health of the skin; too
         much can be toxic; RDA is 5000 IU's taken
         internally, optimal range is 10,000-25,000 IU's; see
         nutrient additives.

S   <u>Vitamin B2</u> - important for healthy tissues and skin;
         see nutrient additives.

S   <u>Vitamin B3</u> - increases circulation; helpful for skin
         rashes; see nutrient additives.

S   <u>Vitamin B6</u> - helpful for skin disorders; see nutrient
         additives.

S   <u>Vitamin C</u> – antioxidant; preservative; can enhance
         mineral absorption, can inhibit nitrosamine
         formation; may be corn based; see nutrient additives.

S   <u>Vitamin C palmitate</u> - see ascorbic acid, nutrient
         additives.

S   <u>Vitamin D</u> - may be helpful to the skin; high doses
         taken internally can be toxic; see nutrient additives.

S   <u>Vitamin E</u> - antioxidant; heals and protects skin; see nutrient additives.

S   <u>Vitamin E acetate</u> - antioxidant; see vitamin E, nutrient additives.

S   <u>Vitamin E linoleate</u> - antioxidant, moisturizer; see vitamin E, nutrient additives.

†S   <u>Wheat germ oil</u>

S   <u>Wild geranium oil</u> – antiseptic; anti-inflammatory.

S   <u>Wild pansy extract</u> – astringent; analgesic.

C   <u>Wild tansy oil</u> – essential oil; anti-bacterial; anti-viral; anti-fungal; toxic if taken internally; use externally with great caution; avoid if pregnant, epileptic; see essential oils.

C1   <u>Wild thyme oil</u> - essential oil; antiseptic; mucous membrane irritant; avoid if pregnant.

C   <u>Wild yam extract</u> - CIR panel says insufficient data to support safety.

C   <u>Wintergreen oil</u> – see methyl salicylate.

CA   <u>Witch hazel</u> – herb; anti-inflammatory; astringent; skin irritant; see ethyl alcohol.

X   <u>Wood alcohol</u> - see methyl alcohol.

*C   <u>Xanthan gum</u> – may cause eye and skin irritation; potentially harmful if absorbed through skin, inhaled or ingested; extracted with toxic organic solvents; solvent residue may remain in the product; contains "approved" levels of lead and arsenic; not adequately tested.

C   <u>Xanthene</u> – interferes with cellular activity; may cause acne.

X   <u>Xylene</u> – skin and eye irritant; toxic if inhaled or ingested; neurotoxin; possible teratogen; carcinogenicity needs to be investigated; not adequately tested.

C1   <u>Yarrow extract</u> - CIR panel says insufficient data to support safety; see yarrow oil.

C1   <u>Yarrow oil</u> – essential oil; antiseptic; anti-inflammatory; frequent use may cause contact sensitization; use cautiously or avoid if pregnant; see essential oils.

CA   <u>Yellow No. 5 Lake</u> – see FD&C Yellow No. 5 Lake.

CA   <u>Yellow No. 6 Lake</u> - see FD&C Yellow No. 6 Lake.

XA   <u>Yellow No. 11</u> – see D&C yellow No. 11.

S   <u>Ylang ylang oil</u> - essential oil; antiseptic; may cause nausea or headache in concentrated form; frequent use may cause contact sensitization; see essential oils.

φS   <u>Zinc oxide</u> – eye and skin irritant; avoid if dry skin; toxic if swallowed.

†C   <u>Zinc phenolsulfate</u> – skin irritant; adversely affected liver, brain and testes in lab animals; contains ammonium salts, see ammonia.

S   <u>Zingiber officinale</u> – see ginger oil.

C   <u>Zirconium chlorohydrate</u> – skin irritant.

C   <u>Zirconyl chloride</u> – skin irritant; moderately toxic if swallowed.

Choosing Safe Products

Products are classified here according to the ingredients that appeared on the label at the time they were evaluated. These are relative categories designed to guide you to the safer choices on the market. They do not guarantee 100% safety. When choosing a product from this list, compare the ingredients on the label with the cosmetic ingredients listed in this book. You must decide for yourself if the safety of the ingredients in the products you choose measure up to the standards of safety you want for yourself.

The products on this list were evaluated for their potential to cause

- **contact dermatitis** – based upon ingredients they contain that cause allergies, irritation and sensitization,
- **cancer** – based upon ingredients that are carcinogens or have the potential to form carcinogens when combined with other ingredients in the product.

They were not evaluated for ingredients that may contain carcinogenic contaminants or for other adverse reactions. There are many ingredients that may be contaminated with cancer-causing chemicals. Some of the potentially contaminated ingredients include lanolin, PEG, polysorbate 60, sodium laureth-5 sulfate and steareth-30. By checking each ingredient on the label with the ingredients listed in this book, you will be able to identify the others. In addition, manufacturers sometimes change the ingredients in a product, so it is wise to check the label before you decide to buy, each time you buy a product.

The products are classified as:

   This is the safest category.

These products, though considered comparatively safe, may contain aluminum, ammonia compounds, or some ingredients that are irritants, neurotoxins or cause estrogenic effects.

These products, though still considered reasonably safe, have a little higher risk of causing contact dermatitis or containing carcinogenic ingredients, and they may contain aluminum, ammonia compounds, or some ingredients that are irritants, neurotoxins or cause estrogenic effects.

Just because one brand is listed in a particular category doesn't mean that the entire line falls into that category or is even recommended. Some of the other products with that brand name may contain harmful ingredients.

These were the safest products that were evaluated. But it does not mean they are the only "safe" products to choose from. You may find other "safe" products by using this book and reading labels when you are shopping. It also doesn't mean that you won't react to the products on this list. Everyone is a unique individual and there may be an ingredient or combination of ingredients that are generally safe, but they may cause a reaction in you. The fewer the number of ingredients in a product, the less likely a reaction is to occur.

In each category, all the products classified as 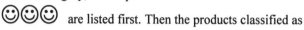 are listed first. Then the products classified as are listed next. The products classified as are listed last.

Many of these products are not found in the typical

department store, grocery store, or pharmacy. Here's some places to look for these products:

- Natural Food Stores
- Health Food Stores
- Food Co-Ops
- Mail-Order Health Catalogs
- Internet

If you are unable to find the products in the ☺☺☺ list or the price is out of your budget, the products in the ☺☺ or ☺ lists may be good alternatives to the more harmful products you may now be using.

Remember: Always read the label before you buy, even for the products on the ☺☺☺ list!

MAKEUP

Foundations

Bare Escentuals
- Beginning & Finishing Powders
- Bronzing & Contouring Powders
- Rice Powder—Pink
- Rice Powder—White

Dr. Hauschka
- Catechu Day Cream (Dark Foundation Color)
- Day Cosmetic (Bronze)
- Ratanhia Day Cream (Medium Foundation Color)

Aubrey Natural Translucent Base
Ida Grae Crème Foundation
Logona
- Tinted Day Cream Beige-Gold
- Tinted Day Cream Beige Rose
Paul Penders Make-Up Cream

Almay Moisture Tint Sports Formula
Clinique Pore-Minimizer Makeup
Cover Girl Clarifying Make-up
Max Factor
- New Definition Make-up
- Pan-Stik Ultra Creamy Make-up
Physician's Formula Le Velvet Film Make-up

Face Powders

Bare Escentuals
- Beginning & Finishing Powders
- Blushing & Highlighting Powders
- Bronzing & Contouring Powders
- Glimmer Powders

Aubrey Silken Earth Make-Up Powder
- Deep Tone
- Light Tone
- Medium
- Rose Tone

Corn Silk Oil Absorbent
- Loose Powder
- Pressed Powder

Ida Grae Translucent Powder
Logona Translucent Powder
Rachel Perry Chamomile Translucent Powder
Revlon Springwater Pressed Powder

Blushes

Bare Escentuals
- Beginning & Finishing Powders
- Blushing & Highlighting Powders
- Bronzing & Contouring Powders
- Glimmer Powders

Dr. Hauschka
- Burgundy Cheek & Lip (Red)
- Rose Cheek & Lip (Pink)
- Cheek & Lip (Apricot)

Ecco Bella Eyeshadow/Blush
Ida Grae Crème Rouge

Paul Penders Blushers

Ida Grae
- Earth Rouge
- Translucent Powder

Maybelline
- Advanced Color Fresh Formula Natural Bristle Brush
- Brush/Blush III Advanced Color Fresh Formula
- Shine Free Oil ControlBlush

Rachel Perry Earth Blush

Concealers

La Formule Aromatherapy Blemish Pen

Cover Girl Replenishing Concealer
Logona Concealer Pen

Lipsticks, Glosses and Lip Pencils

Aubrey Natural Lips
- Natural Red
- Petal Pink
- Mocha Brown
- Crystal Clear

Burt's Beeswax
- Lip Balm
- Lifeguard's Choice Weatherproofing Lip Balm for Sun & Snow

Hemp Balm
- Lemon lime
- Natural
- Spearmint
- Tangerine

Nanak's Lip Smoothee
- Almond
- Coconut
- Spearmint
- Unscented

MoistStic Natural Lip Protection with Tea Tree Oil

Bare Escentuals Conditioning Lip Glaze
Burt's Bees Lip Balm
Dr. Hauschka Lipsticks
Ecco Bella Lip Colors
Ida Grae Earth Lip Crème
Kiss My Face Kiss Colors
Logona Lip Pencils (all colors)
Paul Penders Lip Colors

Bonne Bell Lip Smacker Flavored Lip Gloss
- Bubble Gum
- Peppermint
- Strawberry

Eye Shadows

Bare Escentuals Matte Eyeshadows
Beauty Without Cruelty Eye Color Crayon
Ecco Bella Eyeshadow/Blush
Ida Grae Earth Eyes

Dr. Hauschka Eye Shadow
- Saphir (blue)
- Smaragd (green)
- Topaz (beige)

Ida Grae Earth Eye/Lip Cream
Nature Cosmetics Eyeshadow Pencil
Paul Penders Eye Shadows & Blushers
Pavion Wet 'n' Wild

Almay
- 8-House Eye Color
- Eye Color Single
- Matte Classic Duo

Logona Cosmetic Eye Pencils
L'Oréal Couleur
Max Factor Visual Eyes
Maybelline Blooming Colors Eye Shadow

Monteil Rich Powder Eye Shadow Grand Duo
Nature Cosmetics Brow Liner Pencil
Rachel Perry Eye Shadow

Mascaras

Ecco Bella Mascara
Logona Mascara
- blue
- black
- brown

Chanel Cils Magiques Aqua Resistant Instant Waterproof
Mascara
La prairie Mascara Cellulaire Cellular Mascara
Nature Cosmetics Waterproof Mascara
Paul Penders Mascara
Reviva Liquid Mascara

Almay Longest Lashes Mascara
Bare Escentuals Mascara
Cover Girl Long & Lush Mascara
Estée Lauder
- Luscious Crème Mascara
- More Than Mascara Moisture-Binding Formula
Flame Glow Mascara

HAIR CARE

Shampoos

Bindi Hair Wash
Earth Science Hair Treatment Shampoo
Ginesis Shampoo
Logona

- Extra Care Shampoo
  - Algae
  - Honey & Wheat Germ
- Regular-Care Shampoo
  - Chamomile & Lemon
  - Henna
  - Marigold
  - Nettles
  - Rosemary
- Avocado & Neem Shampoo
- Color-Care Shampoo
- Men's Shampoo & Shower Gel

Mera Shampoo

- Dry Hair
- Normal Hair
- Oily Hair

Thursday Plantation

- Dry Hair Shampoo
- Normal/Oily Hair Shampoo

Urtekram

- Camomile Shampoo
- Desert Moments Shampoo
- Gypsy Night Dream Shampoo
- Ocean Mist Shampoo

Aubrey

- Blue Chamomile Shampoo
- Chamomile Luxurious Herbal Shampoo
- Egyptian Henna Shampoo
- Island Naturals Island Butter Shampoo
- J.A.Y. Desert Herb Shampoo
- Mandarin Magic Ginko Leaf & Earth Smoke Shampoo
- Men's Stock Ginseng Shampoo
- Polynatural 60/80 Hair Rejuvenating Shampoo
- Primrose & Lavender Herbal Shampoo
- QBHL Qillaya Bark Hair Lather
- Rosa Mosqueta Rose Hip Herbal Shampoo
- Saponin A.A.C. Therapeutic Shampoo
- Selenium Natural Blue Shampoo
- Swimmer's Shampoo

Desert Essence Tea Tree Oil Shampoo
Earth Preserv Shampoo (all scents; JC Penney)
Earth Science Herbal Astringent Shampoo
Ecco Bella Wake-Me-Up Shampoo
Faith in Nature Rosemary Shampoo
Nature's Gate Herbal Hair Shampoo
Paul Penders

- Jasmine Chamomile Shampoo
- Peppermint Hops Shampoo
- Rosemary Lavender Shampoo
- Walnut Oil Shampoo

Urtekram Rose & Jasmine Shampoo Soft Highlights

Faith in Nature Shampoo

- Aloe Vera
- Jojoba
- Seaweed

Head Pure & Basic Lite Shampoo
Ivory Shampoo
- Dry/Permed Hair
- Fine Hair
- Mild Formula
- Normal Hair
- Normal to Oily Hair

Jhirmack
- Lite Frequent Use Shampoo For All Hair Types
- Salon E.F.A. moisturizing Shampoo For Dry, Permed & Color Treated Hair

Dandruff Shampoos

Ecco Bella Dandruff Therapy Shampoo

Conditioners

Aubrey Jojoba Oil
Burt's Bees Avocado Butter Hair Treatment
Earth Preserv Hair Vitalizer (all scents; JC Penney)
Faith in Nature Seaweed Conditioner
Ginesis Conditioner
Logona Burdock Root Hair Treatment
Mera Conditioner
- Normal Hair
- Oily Hair

Weleda Conditioner
- Rosemary (with Natural Fragrance)
- Chamomile (with Natural Fragrance)

Aloegen Biotreatment 22 Conditioner
Aubrey Biotin

- Hair Repair
- GPB Glycogen Protein Balancer
- Island Naturals Island Spice Cream Rinse
- Jojoba & Aloe Hair Rejuvenator & Conditioner
- Polynatural 60/80 Hair rejuvenating Conditioner
- Rosa Mosqueta Rose Hip Conditioning Hair Cream
- Rosemary & Sage Hair & Scalp Rinse

Beauty Without Cruelty Oil-Free Extra Body Conditioner
Beehive Botanicals Moisturizing Conditioner
Biopure Conditioner

- Apple with Pectin
- Jojoba

Desert Essence Jojoba Conditioner
Earth Science Conditioner

- Citresoft
- Fragrance Free
- Intensicare

Ecco Bella 60 Second Conditioner
Golden Lotus Rosemary & Lavender Conditioner
Infinity Conditioning Rinse

- Chamomile
- Rosemary

Jason Keratin Conditioner
Logona Rosemary Conditioner
Naturade Aloe Vera Conditioner
Nature's Gate Conditioner

- Biotin
- Jojoba
- Keratin
- Rainwater

Nirvana

- Cherry Bark/Almond Hair Conditioner
- Rosemary/Mint Hair Rinse

Paul Penders
- Lemon Yarrow Cream Rinse Conditioner
- Color Conditioners

Rainbow Research Henna & Biotin Conditioner

Stony Brook Oil-Free Conditioner
- Scented with Natural Fragrance
- Unscented

Unicure Jojoba Hair & Skin Conditioner

Agree Pro-Vitamin (Extra Body & Regular)

Aloegen
- Biogenic Treatment Conditioner
- Biogenic Perm Conditioner
- Tangle-Free Spray-On Conditioner

Aloe Vera – Real Aloe Company Hair Conditioner

Aubrey Swimmer's Condition

Aussie Instant Daily Conditioner with Australian Sea Vegetable Extracts

Beauty Without Cruelty Oil-Free Conditioner

Chica Bella
- Costa Rican Honey
- Herbal Forest
- Monteverde Aloe Vera
- Rare Orchid
- Tropical Bird of Paradise
- Wild Caribbean Seaweed

Earth & Body Vitamin Family Conditioner

Earth Science Herbal Astringent Conditioner

Emerald Forest Conditioner

Faith in Nature Conditioner
- Aloe Vera
- Jojoba
- Rosemary

Finesse Conditioner
- Extra Moisturizing for Dry or Overstyled Hair

- Regular for Normal Hair

Giovanni
- Direct Conditioner-White
- Morebody-Blue
- Nutrafixx-Yellow
- 50/50 Balanced Remoisturizer-Green

Head
- Original Conditioner
- Pure & Basic Lite Conditioning Rinse

Ivory Conditioner
- Dry/Permed Hair
- Fine Hair
- Normal Hair

Jason Conditioner
- Biotin
- EFA Primrose Oil
- Herbal
- Jojoba
- Sea Kelp
- Vitamin E

Jhirmack E.F.A. Moisturizing Conditioner (Dry, Permed & Color Treated Hair)

Kiss My Face Conditioner

L'Oréal Ultra Rich Conditioner
- Extra Body
- Normal

Nature's Gate Awapuhi Conditioner

Pantene
- Progressive Treatment Crème Conditioner de Pantene Extra Body Fine Hair Thickening Formula
- Pro-V Pro-Vitamin Treatment Conditioner
  - Deep Conditioning
  - Regular

Paul Penders German Herbal Hair Repair

Perma Soft Conditioner
- Body Building

- Deep Moisturizing

Prell Conditioner
- Balanced Formula for Normal Hair
- Moisturizing Formula for Dry, Damaged Hair

Reviva Seaweed Conditioner

Salon Selectives Conditioner
- Type F Fortifying
- Type H Highlighting
- Type M Moisturizing
- Type S Sheer
- Type L Leave-On Treatment

Shi Kai Conditioner
- Amla
- Henna Gold
- Moisture Plus
- Spray-On

Suave
- Extra Gentle Conditioner
- Full Body Conditioner
- Perm & Color
- Salon Formula Conditioner Nourishing Formula with Vitamins

Thick Stuff Through & Through Conditioner

Thursday Plantation Tea Tree Conditioner

Trader Joe's Natural Herbal Conditioner

Tropical Botanicals Rainflowers Conditioner

Vidal Sassoon Deep Moisturizing Conditioner

White Rain Conditioner
- Extra Body
- Regular

Women's Hair Coloring Products

Igora Botanic
Logona

- Henna Black
- Henna Natural Red
- Henna Flame Red
- Mahogany
- Sahara
- Walnut Brown

Rainbow Research Henna

Salon Formula Sun-In

Men's Hair Coloring Products

No safe men's hair coloring products were found among the products evaluated. Men should use the women's hair coloring products listed above.

Hair Sprays & Styling Products

Alexandra Avery Hair Oil
Aubrey

- Ginkgo Leaf & Ginseng Root Jelly
- Ginseng Hair Control
- Natural Missst Herbal Hair Spray

Naturade

- Nonalcohol Styling Spray
- Hair Spray with Jojoba

Weleda Rosemary Hair Oil

Aubrey
- Chestnut Brown Natural Body Highliter Mousse
- Design Gel
- Golden Chamomile Natural Body Highliter Mousse
- Soft Black Natural Body Highliter Mousse

Earth Preserv

Earth Science Silk Forte Hair Styling Mist

Alberto VO5
- Conditioning Hard to Hold Nonaerosol Hair Spray
- Extra Body Hard to Hold Nonaerosol Hair Spray
- Hard to Hold Nonaerosol Hair Spray
- Unscented Hard to Hold Nonaerosol Hair Spray
- With Cholesterol Damaged Hair Treatment

Aloegen
- Hair Sculpting Setting Gel
- Styling Spritz
- Hair Spray

Aquanet Nonaerosol Hair Spray
- Extra Super Hold
- Regular Hold
- Super Hold
- Unscented Regular Hold
- Unscented Super Hold

Aussie
- Mega Styling Nonaerosol Spray
  - Aussie Sprunch Spray
  - Ultra Firm Working Spray
- Scould Spray Gel Nonaerosol Professional Sculpting & Molding Hair Fixture

Clairol Final Net Nonaerosol Hair Spray
- Extra Hold

- Ultimate Hold

Earth Science Silk Lite Hair Styling Mist

Finesse Nonaerosol Hairspray (Extra Hold)

Giovanni

- Sunset Sculpset Lavender
- Vitapro Fusion-Orange
- L.A. Hold Black
- L.A. Natural Red
- Natural Mousse

Jhirmack Nonaerosol Hairspray

Mera

- Hair Spray
- Misting Gel

Rave Nonaerosol

- Hair Spray
    - Extra Hold
    - Super Hold
    - Ultra Hold
- All in One Hair Spray with Conditioning Nutrients
    - Natural Hold
    - Super Hold
    - Ultra Hold

Salon Selectives (10 Extra Hold)

Shi Kai

- Extra Hold Finishing Spray
- Super Hold Styling Spray

Style Nonaerosol Hair Spray

- Super Hold
- Unscented Super Hold

Suave Nonaerosol Hair Spray (Extra Hold)

White Rain Nonaerosol Hair Spray

- Dry or Treated Hair
- Extra Hold
- Unscented Extra Hold

Men's Hair Sprays & Styling Products

Alexandra Avery Hair Oil

Aloegen
- Hair Sculpting Setting Gel
- Styling Spritz

Consort
- Fine Mist Pump Hair Spray
  - Extra Hold
  - Unscented
- Pump Hair Spray Super Hold Spritz

The Dry Look Pump Hair Spray (Max Hold)

Vaseline Hair Tonic and Scalp Conditioner

Toothpastes & Powders

Auromere Toothpaste
Beehive Botanicals Propolis Toothpaste
Bioforce Echinacea
Desert Essence Tea Tree Oil Toothpaste
Herbal –Vedic Herbal Toothpaste
Home Health
- Peri-Dent Herbal Gum Massage
- Salt 'N Soda Toothpowder
Logona Toothpaste
- Peppermint & Clay
- Rosemary & Sage
Mer-Flu-An
- Anise Toothpowder
- Cinnamon & Mint Toothpaste
- Lemon Lime Toothpowder
- Peppermint Toothpowder
Nature's Gate Toothpaste
- Cherry Gel
- Crème de Anise
- Crème de Peppermint
- Mint Gel
- Wintergreen Gel
Peelu
- Toothpaste
- Toothpowder
Rainbow Research Mint Toothpaste
Tom's of Maine Toothpaste (nonfluoride)
- Propolis & Myrrh/ Cinnamint
- Propolis & Myrrh/ Fennel
- Propolis & Myrrh/ Spearmint
Vicco Pure Herbal Toothpaste

Weleda
- Plant Toothpaste
- Pink Toothpaste
- Salt & Soda Toothpaste

Xylifresh Toothpaste
- Cinnamon
- Peppermint
- Spearmint

Mouthwashes

Desert Essence Tea Tree Mouthwash
Logona
- Cistacea Oral Spray
- Herbal Mouthwash Concentrate

Merfluan Mouthwash Concentrate
Tom's Mouthwash
- Cinnamint
- Spearmint

Weleda Mouthwash
Xylifresh Mouthwash

FEMININE HYGIENE

Feminine Deodorants, Douches & Hygiene Preparations

Bee Kind Disposable Douche
Bio Botanica Douche Concentrate
Camo Care Disposable Douche
Massengill
- All Natural Extra Mild Vinegar & Water No Additives Disposable Douche
- Baking Soda & Water Disposable Douche
- Natural Ingredients Extra Cleansing with Pura Clean Disposable Douche
Summer's Eve Disposable Douche Vinegar & Water

Summer's Eve
- Feminine Powder
- Fresh Scent
- Herbal Freshness Disposable Douche
- Hint of Musk Disposable Douche
Vagisil Feminine Powder

Note: Frequent douching is not advisable. It may increase the risk for cervical cancer.

Organically grown cotton pads

Note:
- Tampons may be contaminated with carcinogens and are associated with Toxic Shock Syndrome, which is potentially fatal. High-absorbency tampons left in for prolonged periods or overnight increase the risk.
- Bleached cotton pads may be contaminated with carcinogens.

NAIL PRODUCTS

Nail Polishes, Hardeners & Protectors

De Lore

- Chip Proof
- Nail Fix
- Nail Protector

De Lore Nail Hardener

Note:
- The nails are porous and will absorb the chemicals in the nail products.
- Nail products are hazardous to children and may cause poisoning.

Even though the above nail products are relatively safe compared to other nail products, I do not recommend the use of nail polishes, hardeners or protectors. If your nails are soft, weak, chip or are otherwise unhealthy, it is a sign of improper nutrition or ill health. Correct the underlying nutritional or health problem and your nails will become healthy naturally.

SKIN PRODUCTS

Deodorants & Antiperspirants

Desert Essence Tea Tree Roll-on Deodorant
Earth Science Liken Deodorant (Unscented)
Fabergé Power Stick Antiperspirant & Deodorant (Unscented)
Home Health Roll-on Deodorant (Unscented)
Jason Deodorant Apricot & E Stick
Lady Speed Stick Antiperspirant & Deodorant (No Dyes or Fragrance)
Lavilin
- Foot Deodorant
- Underarm Deodorant
Le Crystal Naturel Deodorant
Logona
- Deodorant
- Roll-on Deodorant
Mitchum Super Dry Roll-on Antiperspirant & Deodorant (Unscented)
Secret Roll-on Antiperspirant & Deodorant (Unscented)
Speed Stick Antiperspirant & Deodorant Super Dry (Unscented)
Suave Stick Antiperspirant & Deodorant (Unscented)
Thursday Plantation Roll-on Deodorant
Weleda Deodorant
- Citrus
- Sage

Almay Antiperspirant Solid Deodorant Unscented
Bellmira Deodorant
CamoCare Deodorant
Canoe Deodorant Stick

Jason Deodorant
- Tea Tree Roll-on
- Tea Tree Stick

Nature De France Stick Deodorant
- Floral Scent
- Gardenia Scent
- Herbal Scent
- Unscented

Queen Helene Vitamin E Deodorant Stick
Tom's of Maine Deodorant
- Stick (All Scents)
- Aloe & Buffered Alum Roll-on
- Aloe & Coriander Roll-on

Ban Roll-On Antiperspirant & Deodorant
- Ocean Breeze
- Unscented

Barth Stick Deodorant
Degree
- Roll-On Antiperspirant & Deodorant
    - Powder Fresh
    - Regular
    - Shower Clean
- Solid Antiperspirant & Deodorant
    - Powder Fresh
    - Regular
    - Shower Clean
    - Sport
    - Unscented

Earth Science Lichen Deodorant
Fabergé Power Stick Antiperspirant & Deodorant
- Active Sport
- Cool Scent
- Musk

- Regular

Five-Day Antiperspirant & Deodorant Pads
Head Green Tea Roll-On Deodorant
Home Health Roll-on Deodorant (Scented)
Irish Spring Solid Antiperspirant & Deodorant

- Morning Breeze
- Sport Fresh

Jason

- Apricot & E Roll-On Deodorant
- Herbs &Spice Roll-On Deodorant

Old Spice

- Antiperspirant & Deodorant Stick (Original)
- Pump Deodorant
  - Classic Sport
  - Fresh
  - Musk
  - Original

Queen Helene

- Aloe Deodorant Stick
- Mint Julep Deodorant

Right Guard Sport Stick

- Antiperspirant & Deodorant
  - Alpine Air
  - Fresh
  - Musk
  - Surf Spray
- Deodorant (Fresh)

Secret Roll-on Antiperspirant & Deodorant

- Fresh
- Regular
- Sporty Clean
- Spring Breeze

Speed Stick Antiperspirant & Deodorant Super Dry

- Classic Scent
- Fresh Scent
- Musk

- Spice Scent

Suave Stick Antiperspirant & Deodorant
- Aloe Fresh
- Baby Powder
- Regular
- Sport
- Unscented

Sure Solid Antiperspirant & Deodorant
- Desert Spice
- Outdoor Fresh
- Powder Dry
- Regular

Teen Spirit
- Roll-on Antiperspirant & Deodorant
  - Baby Powder Soft
  - California Breeze
- Wide Solid Antiperspirant & Deodorant
  - Caribbean Cool
  - Ocean Ssurf
  - Romantic Rose

Tussy
- Cream Deodorant (Powder Fresh)
- Roll-on Antiperspirant & Deodorant

Bath Oils, Bubble Baths & Mineral Baths

Abracadabra
- California Bath
- Foaming Aloe Vera Bath
- Luxury Bubble Bath
- Mineral Bath
- Sport Therapy

Aubrey Eucalyptus Spa Bath

Aura Cacia
- Massage and Bath Oils (all)
- Mineral Bath
  - Deep Heat
  - Energize
  - Heart Song
  - Inspiration
  - Tranquility

Earth Preserv Bath Crystals (all scents; JC Penney)
Ecco Bella Body Soaks
- Detox Foaming
- Dieter's
- Love Foaming
- Sleep Foaming

Faith in Nature Essential Bath Foam
Logona
- Herbal Bubble Bath Refresh
- Bubble BathRelax with Hops-Chamomile

Olbas Bath
Sofie's Botanical Bath Creations (All)
Weleda Bath Oils (all)

Aubrey
- Chamomile Bubble Bath Oil
- Rosa Mosqueta Bath Jaléa
- Relax-R-Bath

Earth Preserv Nourishing Body Bath (all scents; JC Penney)
Paul Penders Calming Flower Bath Oil
Pure Approach
- Seaweed Bubble Bath
- Seaweed Non-Foaming Bath

Calgon
- Bubbling Milk Bath (Powder Fresh with Baby Oil)
- Moisturizing Foam Bath (Powder Fresh with Foaming Milk & Baby Oil)

Jean Naté Sheersilk Bath & Body Oil

Queen Helene Batherapy

Powders for Body Care

Desert Essence Talc Free Body Powder

Jason Body Powder Talc Free
- Aloe Vera 84%
- Tea Tree Oil
- Chamomile

Nutribiotic Natural Body & Foot Powder

Dr. Hauschka Body powder

Note: Talc is a carcinogen. *Never* use talc on babies and children. Use of talcum powder for feminine hygiene increases the risk of ovarian cancer.

Shaving Creams

Paul Penders Lemon Balm Shave Cream

Aubrey Mint & Ginseng Shaving Cream

Logona Men's Shaving Cream

Tom's of Maine Shave Cream

Skin Lotions

Alba Botanica Unscented Very Emollient Body Lotion
Autumn Harp Body Lotion
Body Love Aroma Lotion
Burt's Bees
- Coconut Foot Cream
- Farmer's Market Nutritive Carrot Cream

Chica Bella Cloud Forest Avocado
Enlightened Visions New Moon Nourishing Skin & Nail Salve
Kiss My Face Oil-Free Moisturizer
Pretty Baby Herbal Cream
Paul Penders Oriental Flower Body Lotion
Soft Sense Skin Essentials Skin Lotion (Extra Moisturizing for Dry Skin with Vitamin E)
Trader Joe's Moisturizing Skin Lotion

Alba Botanica Emollient Body Lotion
Aubrey
- Cell Therapy
- Collagen & Almond Oil
- Collagen TCM Therapeutic Cream Moisturizer
- Elastin NMF
- Evening Primrose Complexion & Body Lotion
- Evening Primrose Oil
- Ginseng Face Cream Men's Stock
- Vegacell Herbal Cellular Complex
- Maintenance for Young Skin

117

- Mandarin Magic Moisturizer
- Rejeunesse Moisturizing Cream
- Rosa Mosqueta
  - Hand & Body Lotion
  - Rose Hip Moisturizing Cream
  - Rose Hip Seed Oil
- Vegetal Collagen Moisturizer
- Seaherbal Massage Lotion
- Swimmers Moisturizer

Beauty Without Cruelty Oil Free Moisture Cream
Beehive Botanicals Therapeutic Derma Cream
Curê Moisturizing Cream/Lotion (Fragrance Free)
Desert Essence Jojoba Rosemary Lotion
Earth Science Hand & Body Lotion
Ecco Bella
- Skin Nourishers
  - After Workout
  - Calm Spirit
  - Energy Boost
  - Erotic
  - Farewell Cellulite
  - Tocca Mi
- Skin Facial Nourishers
  - Dry-Mature
  - Normal-Sensitive
  - Oily-Problem
- Natural Moisture Day Cream
- Vanilla Body Lotion

Earth Preserv Skin Moisturizer (all scents; JC Penney)
Home Health
- Skin Lotion
  - Almond
  - Coconut
  - Jasmine
  - Unscented
- Liquid Lanolin

Jacki's Magic Lotion
- Almond
- Lavender
- Orange-Vanilla
- Rose-Mint

Jason Vitamin E Hand & Body Lotion

Logona
- Lotions
  - Almond Body Lotion
  - Free Body Lotion
  - Herbal Blossom Body Lotion
- Creams
  - Almond Extra Care Cream
  - Aloe & Hypericum Cream
  - Avocado Extra Care Cream
  - Carrot Extra Care Cream
  - Free Facial Moisturizing Cream
  - Hand Cream
  - Linden Blossom Extra Care Cream with Vitamin E
  - Mallow & Jojoba Cream
  - Rose & Wheat Germ Cream
  - Rosemary & Chamomile Cream
- Oils
  - Chamomile Bodycare Oil
  - Hypericum Bodycare Oil
  - Marigold Bodycare Oil
  - Massage Oil

Nature's Gate
- Moisturizing Lotion
- Fragrance-Free Moisturizing Lotion
- Skin Therapy Lotion

Shi Kai Fragrance-Free Hand & Body Lotion

Stony Brook Oil-Free Body Lotion (Unscented)

Sunshine ProductsAromassage Lotion
- Refreshing Herbal Magic
- Sensual Bouquet

Beauty Without Cruelty Aloe and E Moisture Cream
Beehive Botanicals
- Honey and Almond Hand & Body Lotion
- Home and Bee Pollen Body Moisturizer
Curê Moisturizing Cream/Lotion
Earth & Body Care Aloe Vera Family Lotion
Jacki's Magic Lotion
- Coconut
- Jasmine
- Rose
Jergens Vitamin E & Lanolin
Keri Lotion Silky Smooth Formula for Soft Skin Everyday
(Fragrance Free)
Kiss My Face
- Fragrance-Free Olive & Aloe Moisturizer
- Honey & Calendula Moisturizer
- Vitamin A & E Moisturizer
Moisturel Lotion
Nivea
- Crème Ultra Moisturizing
- Moisturizing Lotion Extra Enriched Formula
Reviva Elastin Body Lotion
Shi Kai Hand & Body Lotion
- Apricot/Rose
- Cucumber/Melon
Stony Brook Oil-Free Body Lotion (Scented)
Tropical Botanicals Babacu Nut Body Lotion

Soaps

Aubrey Rose Mosqueta Moisturizing Cleansing Bar
Aura Cacia Bath Soap
- Deep Heat
- Energize
- Euphoria Aromatherapy
- Heart Song
- Inspiration
- Tranquility

Barth
- Aloe Vera Soap
- Cocoa Butter Soap
- Lecithin Soap

Bindi Herbal Cleanser
Boraxo Powdered Hand Soap
Brookside Soap
- Oatmeal/Almond
- Spearmint
- Rosemary/Lavender
- Cinnamon
- Extra Mild Herbal
- Extra Mild Unscented
- Lemongrass/Lime
- Lime

Burt's Bees Orange Essence Facial Cleanser
Calben Pure Soap
Chandrika Soap
Clearly Natural Glycerine Bar
Chica Bella
- Bird of Paradise
- Costa Rican Honey
- Deep Earth Clay
- Deep Sea Algae
- Honey Jasmine

- Monteverde Aloe Vera
- Organic Orange Peel
- Rare Orchid

Dr. Bronner's Pure Castile Soap
- Liquid
  - Almond
  - Eucalyptus
  - Lavender
  - Peppermint
  - Tea Tree
- Bar
  - Lemon
  - Rose

Earth Preserv
- Cream Soaps (all; JC Penney)
- Glycerine Soaps (all; JC Penney)

Faith in Nature Bar Soap
- Lavender
- Orange
- Pine
- Rosemary

Kiss My Face
- Soap
- Olive & Aloe Soap
- Olive & Herbal Soap

Logona
- Body Soaps
  - Chamomile
  - Herbal
  - Honey & Marigold
- Cistacea Intensive Cleansing Lotion
- Free Soap

Nature De France Soaps
- Algoli
- Argile
- Argile Blanche

- Argile Rose
- Argimiel

Nature Works Herbal Soap
- Balm
- Chamomile
- Lavender
- Marigold
- Rosemary

Pretty Baby Herbal Soap Shampoo & Body Bar
Pure Approach
- Clay Soaps
- Combination Skin Soap
- Dry Skin Soap
- Emile Soaps
  - Honey
  - Olive/Lavender
  - Passion Fruit
  - Vanilla
- Loofa Soap
- Sea Mud Soap
- Sensitive Skin Soap
- Shea Butter Soap

Reviva Aloe Chamomile Soap
Sirena Coconut Soap
Weleda
- Iris Soap
- Rose Soap
- Rosemary Soap

Alexandra Avery
- Wild Mountain Herbs Soap
- Jungle Blossoms Soap

Cashmere Bouquet Soap
Home Health Palma Christi Cleansing Bar

Logona Facial Scrub Cream
NutriBiotic Nonsoap Skin Cleanser
Pure Approach Emile's Honey Shower Gel
Rainbow Research
- Aloe/Oatmeal Bar
- Clay Cleansing Bar
Sirena Vitamin E Soap
Zest

Aloe Vera – Real Aloe Company Aloe Vera Soap
Barth Soaps
- Cocoa Butter
- Lecithin
Caress Body Bar
Dove
- Pink Beauty Bar
- Unscented
- White
Eastern Star Soap
Head
- Green Tea Deodorant Soap
- Lotus Body Scrub Bar
Kappus
- Cream Soaps
- Glycerine Soaps
Pond's Cold Crème
Reviva
- Honey & Almond Scrub
- Oatmeal Soap
San Francisco Soap Company Soaps (all)
Sappo Hill Glycerine Crème Soap
Softsoap Sensitive Skin Cleansing Liquid

OUTDOOR PRODUCTS

Sunscreens

Aubrey Organics
- Nature Tan 100% Natural Tanning Cream Light Protection Formula SPF 8
- Rosa Mosqueta Sun Protection Herbal Butter SPF 15
- Saving Face SPF 15 Natural Sunblock Protection Spray
- Sunshade 15 100% Natural Sunscreen Cream SPF 15
- Titania SPF 25 Full Spectrum Natural Herbal Sunblock
- Ultra 15 Natural Herbal Sunblock

Insect Repellants

All TerrainNatural Herbal Armor Insect Repellant Pump Spray No DEET
Green Ban for People Herbal Insect Repellant & Itch Soother
Natrapel
- Lotion
- Pump spray

BABIES & CHILDREN

Shampoos

Aubrey Organics Natural Baby & Kids Shampoo
Ginesis Chemical Free Baby Shampoo

California Baby Botanical Shampoo and Bodywash
Urtekram Children's Shampoo

Healthy Times Baby's Herbal Garden Pansy Flower Shampoo
Rainbow Shampoo for Kids
Tom's Natural Baby Shampoo

Conditioners

California Baby Botanical
- Hair Conditioner
- Hair Detangler

Healthy Times Baby's Herbal Garden Chamomile Blossom
Conditioner

Rainbow Detangler for kids

Baby Powders

Burt's Bees Baby Bee Dusting Powder Talc Free
Country Comfort Baby Powder
Desitin Cornstarch Baby Powder
Diaparene Cornstarch Baby Powder
Johnson's Baby Powder Cornstarch
Johnson's Baby, Medicated
Magick Baby Fragrance-Free Powder
Nutra Soothe Medicated
Velvet Fresh Powder

Note: Talc is a carcinogen. *Never* use talc on babies and children.

Lotions and Creams

Burt's Bees Baby Bee
- Skin Cream
- Diaper Ointment with Vitamin A & E

Gaia's Children's Skin Cream for Baby Bottoms
Healthy Times Baby's Herbal Garden Sunflower Petal Baby Oil

California Baby Botanical Moisturizing Cream
Country Comfort Baby Cream
Flanders Buttocks
Healthy Times Baby's Herbal Garden Sweet Violet Lotion
Weleda
- Baby Cream
- Diaper Care

Soaps

Dr. Bronner's Aloe Vera Baby Mild Pure Castile Soap
Healthy Times Baby's Herbal Garden
- Sunflower Baby Bar
- Aloe & Chamomile Baby Bar
Weleda Calendula Baby Soap

Bubble Baths

California Baby Herbal Chamomile Bubble Bath

Abracadabra Kid's Bubble Bath
Mr. Bubble Bath Powder
Rainbow Bubble Bath for Kids
Sesame Street Bubble Bath Powder

Toothpastes

Logona Children's Toothpaste
Tom's of Maine (nonfluoride) Children's Toothpaste

Sunscreens

Aubrey Organics Green Tea Sunblock for Children

If the products you use aren't on this list, check the ingredients with the ingredients listed in this book to see if the ingredients meet your personal safety standards. You may also want to check to see if they are listed in *The Safe Shopper's Bible* by David Steinman and Samuel Epstein, M. D. (see references). This book has an extensive list of products rated as *Little to No Risk, Minimal Risk* and *Caution.* It lists products that are recommended as well as those that are not recommended because of their high potential to cause contact dermatitis or contain carcinogenic ingredients.

Glossary

Allergen – may cause allergic or hypersensitivity reaction.

Antibacterial –destroys bacteria or suppresses their growth; used in treating infections, preserving food and cosmetics.

Antidandruff – prevents excess dandruff formation.

Anti-inflammatory – suppresses inflammation; reduces pain, heat, redness and swelling resulting from injury or infection.

Antimicrobial – kills microorganisms or suppresses their growth; used in preserving food and cosmetics.

Antioxidant – prevents oxidation, protects against free radicals and slows cell and tissue damage.

Astringent – causes the tissues to contract.

Carcinogen – causes cancer.

Carrier oil – an oil used to dilute pure essential oils.

Cheilitis – inflammation of the lips.

CIR – Cosmetic Ingredient Review, an independent panel established by the Cosmetic, Toiletry and Fragrance Association (CTFA) in 1976 to review and assess the safety of ingredients used in cosmetics.

Colorant – color additive

Contact dermatitis – a skin reaction that occurs after exposure to a substance that either irritates your skin or causes an allergic response.

Contact sensitization - a delayed allergic reaction resulting in allergic contact dermatitis.

Dermatitis – inflammation of the skin.

Essence – scent; solution of a volatile oil in alcohol.

Essential oil – natural, aromatic oils distilled from plants; volatile oils.

FDA approved colorant – color additives that the FDA has approved for use in food and cosmetics.

GRAS (Generally Recognized As Safe) – food additives that were in use before 1958 and were considered safe, even if they had never been tested; between 1958 and 1997, manufacturers had to submit a petition to the FDA for approval of a new food additive; in 1997, the FDA decided to let the manufacturers decide if an additive is GRAS and no longer required premarket approval.

Herbs – plants, including leaves, bark, berries, roots, gums, seeds, stems and flowers that have been used for thousands of years to help maintain good health;. may use harmful chemicals to extract the herbs or may use the herbs in concentrations too low to be of benefit; may cause adverse reactions or may be very beneficial.

Humectant – a substance which moistens or dilutes.

Irritant – causes irritation.

Mutagen – causes genetic changes and may lead to cancer or hereditary diseases.

Natural emollient – softening or soothing substance derived from natural sources.

Natural emulsifier – a substance derived from natural sources that causes oil and water to mix and form a stable mixture.

Natural preservatives – protect against the growth of microorganisms which cause spoilage in food and cosmetics, but have a limited shelf life compared to chemical preservatives which are added in large enough quantities to yield a 2 – 3 year shelf life.

Neurotoxic – poisonous or destructive to nerve tissue.

Neurotoxin – a substance that is poisonous or destructive to nerve tissue.

Nitrosating agents – chemical compounds classified as secondary amines, including DEA, MEA, TEA, that combine with nitrogen-containing compounds to form nitrosamines.

Nitrosamines – chemical compounds formed when secondary amines combine with nitrites. Most nitrosamines are carcinogenic.

OSHA - Occupational Safety & Health Administration in the US Department of Labor.

Photosensitivity – increased reaction of the skin to sunlight; may burn more easily; when using ingredients that cause photosensitivity, avoid direct sunlight for up to 12 hours.

Phototoxic chemical – harmless chemical, synthetic or natural, used in sunscreens which becomes toxic and causes adverse reactions due to biochemical reaction with UV rays of the sun

Phototoxicity – being phototoxic.

Preservatives – protect against the growth of microorganisms which cause spoilage in food and cosmetics.

Sensitizer – causes the body to react more strongly to a substance.

Sunscreen – protects against some or all of the harmful rays of the sun.

Surfactants – water soluble compounds that lower the surface tension of water allowing it to spread more easily; soaps, emulsifying agents.

Synthetic emollient – softening or soothing substance derived from synthetic chemicals; most cause adverse skin reactions.

Synthetic emulsifier – a substance derived from synthetic chemicals that causes oil and water to mix and form a stable mixture; most cause adverse reactions.

Synthetic humectant – synthetic moisturizers; many cause adverse reactions.

Teratogen – causes birth defects.

Vitamin – a substance naturally occurring in food that is necessary for normal metabolic functioning of the body.

REFERENCES

Botanical Dermatology Database. http://bodd.web.cf.ac.uk/

Britton, Jade & Tamara Kircher, The Complete Book of Home Herbal Remedies. Buffalo, New York: Firefly Books, 1998.

Bunney, Sarah, Editor, The Illustrated Book of Herbs; Their Medicinal and Culinary Uses. New York: Gallery Books, 1984.

Castleman, Michael, The Healing Herbs. Emmaus, PA: Rodale Press, 1991.

Center For Science in the Public Interest, http://www.cspinet.org

Chevallier, Andrew, The Encyclopedia of Medicinal Plants. New York: DK Publishing, Inc., 1996.

Dorland's Illustrated Medical Dictionary

Farlow, Christine H., DC, Food Additives: A Shopper's Guide To What's Safe & What's Not. KISS For Health Publishing, 1999.

Farlow, Christine H., DC, Healthy Eating: For Extremely Busy People Who Don't Have Time For It. KISS For Health Publishing, 1998.

FDA Center for Food Safety & Applied Nutrition, http://vm.cfsan.fda.gov/

Gardiner, Anthony, Medicinal Herbs and Essential Oils. Edison, New Jersey: Chartwell Books, Inc., 1995.

Grieve, M., A Modern Herbal. New York; Dover Publications, Inc., 1971. Volumes I and II.

Hampton, Aubrey, Natural Organic Hair and Skin Care. Tampa, Florida: Organica Press, 1987

Higley, Connie and Alan, Reference Guide for Essential Oils. Olathe, KS: Abundant Health, 1998.

Krauss, Beatrice H., Native Plants Used As Medicine in Hawaii.

Lewis, Grace Ross, 1001 Chemicals in Everyday Products, New York: John Wiley & Sons, Inc., 1999

Nonprescription Products: Formulations & Features '96-97. Washington, DC: American Pharmaceutical Association, 1996.

Ody, Penelope, The Complete Medicinal Herbal. New York: Dorling Kindersley, Inc., 1993.

Online Medical Dictionary, http;//www.gralab.ac.uk

Ryman, Daniele, Aromatherapy; The Complete Guide to Plant and Flower Essences for Health and Beauty. New York: Bantam Books, 1993.

Schiller, Carol & David, Aromatherapy Oils: A Complete Guide. New York:Sterling Publishing Co., Inc., 1996.

Sharamon, Shalila and Bodo J. Baginski, The Healing Power of Grapefruit Seed. Lotus Light Publications, 1997

Smeh, Nikolaus J., MS, Health Risks in Today's Cosmetics: The Handbook for a Lifetime of Healthy Skin and Hair. Alliance Publishing Co., 1994.

Stabile, Toni, Everything You Want to Know About Cosmetics. New York: Dodd, Mead & Company, 1984.

Steinman, David & Samuel S. Epstein, M.D., The Safe Shopper's Bible; A Consumer's Guide to Nontoxic Household Products, Cosmetics and Food. New York: Macmillan, 1995

Tenney, Louise, M.H., Today's Herbal Health, Third Edition. Prove, Utah: Woodland Books, 1992.

Tierra, Michael, C.A., N.D., Planetary Herbology. Santa Fe, New Mexico: Lotus Press, 1988.

Truth in Labeling Campaign, http://www.truthinlabeling.org

Vitamins.com, http://www.vitamins.com/encyclopedia

West, Bruce, D.C., Health Alert Newsletter

Wilson, Roberta, The Complete Guide to Understanding & Using Aromatherapy for Vibrant Health & Beauty. New York: Avery Publishing Group, 1995.

Winter, Ruth, A Consumer's Dictionary of Cosmetic Ingredients. New York: Three Rivers Press, 1999.

Books By This Author

DYING TO LOOK GOOD: The Disturbing Truth About What's Really in Your Cosmetics, Toiletries and Personal Care Products
$10.95 + $4.00 S&H + 7.75% tax (CA residents)

FOOD ADDITIVES: A Shopper's Guide To What's Safe & What's Not
$4.95 + $1.50 S&H + 7.75% tax (CA residents)

HEALTHY EATING: For Extremely Busy People Who Don't Have Time For It.
$7.95 + $3.00 S&H + 7.75% tax (CA residents)

When ordering more than one book, the shipping charge is the highest shipping charge + $1.00 for each additional book, i.e. the shipping charge to order all three of the above books is:
$4.00 + $1.00 + $1.00 = $6.00

To order, send check or money order to:

KISS For Health Publishing
P.O. Box 462335-C • Escondido, CA 92046-2335
(760) 735-8101 • Fax (760) 746-8937
e-mail: kiss4health@netscape.net

Q: Which of the following may contain MSG?
   a. shampoo   b. cosmetics   c. yogurt

To find out the truth about how MSG may be affecting your life, send a long self addressed stamped envelope to KISS For Health Publishing at the above address for your free MSG Safety Report

Excerpts, information on the contents of these books and reviews may be found on Amazon.com or at
http://www.ReadersNdex.com/kiss4health
http://www.bookmasters.com/marktplc/00084.htm.